anorexia and bulimia

A PARENTS' GUIDE

D0306624

To my children Joanna, Dominic,
Katie, Amy and Alex

anorexia and bulimia

A PARENTS' GUIDE TO RECOGNISING EATING DISORDERS AND TAKING CONTROL

DR DEE DAWSON

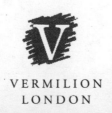

VERMILION
LONDON

1 3 5 7 9 10 8 6 4 2

Text © Dr Dee Dawson 2001

Dr Dee Dawson has asserted her right to be identified as the author of
this work under the Copyright, Designs and Patents Act 1988.

First published in the United Kingdom in 2001 by Vermilion
an imprint of Ebury Press
Random House
20 Vauxhall Bridge Road · London SW1V 2SA

Random House Australia (Pty) Limited
20 Alfred Street · Milsons Point · Sydney · New South Wales 2061 · Australia

Random House New Zealand Limited
18 Poland Road · Glenfield · Auckland 10 · New Zealand

Random House South Africa (Pty) Limited
Endulini · 5A Jubilee Road · Parktown 2193 · South Africa

Random House UK Limited Reg. No. 954009

Papers used by Vermilion are natural,recyclable products made from
wood grown in sustainable forests.

A CIP catalogue record for this book is available from the British Library.

ISBN 0 09 187652 4

Designed by Lovelock & Co.

Printed and bound in Great Britain by Mackays

Although every effort has been made to ensure that the contents of this book are
accurate, it must not be treated as a substitute for qualified medical advice. Always
consult a qualified medical practitioner. Neither the Author nor the Publisher can be
held responsible for any loss or claim arising out of the use, or misuse, of the suggestions made or the failure to take medical advice.

14. NOV. 2002

Contents

Foreword

Before coming to Rhodes Farm I had cheated my way through two different child and adolescent units, I had even managed to lose more weight in one of them.

As soon as I arrived in Rhodes Farm I knew it was different. I could see that I wouldn't be allowed to get away with anything. That didn't stop me trying but you always found out and I always had to catch up. In the end I just gave up and then I had time to think about what I was doing.

I had my ups and downs, I was angry with everyone for making me gain weight but I came through. I had met a brick wall and once I saw there was no way around it I had to climb over.

I never looked back once I left Rhodes Farm and although I didn't show it at the time, I am very grateful for the help you all gave me. Without you I don't know where I'd be now.

Letter from an ex-patient

Preface

At Rhodes Farm we have learnt that the key to success is being firm and consistent. The children know that negotiation and compromise are not words in our vocabulary when it comes to eating. One of my patients once described me as the 'rock in a frock', not a very flattering description but one which depicts the unyielding stance we take with refeeding our young patients. Our role is to help and support parents in being the rock their children need to cling to whilst they and their therapists struggle to overcome their eating disorder.

Since Rhodes Farm opened 10 years ago we have cared for nearly 600 anorexic and bulimic children, the vast majority having been treated for many months or years before coming to us.

Over the years we have been surprised by the number of parents who have never been offered any advice. We are frequently told 'no one ever told us what to do!' Some have even told us 'the doctors asked *us* what *we* thought we should do'.

Parents are in the habit of consulting doctors over less serious childhood ailments and being told exactly how to proceed. It is puzzling, therefore, why parents of anorexic children are left to muddle through with very little practical help.

I was prompted to write this book because we believe that many parents we have seen could have helped their children overcome their problems and may not have needed in-patient treatment if they had had a better understanding of the illness and some concrete advice. Indeed, in many cases, the illness might have been avoided altogether if early warning signs had been spotted. So many parents are told quite early on in their child's illness that they should stand back, not interfere, allow their child to eat what she wants, how much she wants, when she wants and where she wants. While this may be a way of proceeding with adult patients, this approach is exactly the opposite of the one we have used at Rhodes Farm for the last 10 years.

Prevention is better than cure and I will give advice on how to try to prevent children becoming obsessed about their diet. Younger and younger children are experimenting with dieting and worrying about their body shape. I am often asked what one should do about a child who is overweight or who thinks she is and is considering a diet. I will discuss how these issues should be approached.

I will also deal with starvation, bingeing, vomiting, laxative abuse, compulsive exercising and self-harm, talk about why it happens, the long-term consequences and what you should do.

There will be some children who will benefit from an in-patient stay and will not be able to overcome their difficulties without a spell away from home and some intensive family therapy. I will tell you what to look for in a good unit and explain the mysteries of therapy. When a child is discharged from the unit you must be willing and able to support her when she comes home, and I will tell you how best to do this.

You may well want to read this book from cover to cover. I hope you will derive comfort from the fact that the problems you are facing are not unique, and feel empowered by the concrete and practical advice offered. Or you might be seeking help for a specific problem and want to be able to use this as a reference book. You should find your problem or worry clearly described and dealt with. If you are reading cover to cover you may find the occasional issue is dealt with more than once as it is relevant to more than one chapter.

In our many years of dealing with children with eating disorders we have come to realize that not only can the illness affect entire families but that families, especially parents, can play a significant role in the treatment of the illness. As parents you will need support and information, and this book aims to deliver both. It is easy to feel helpless when trying to cope with an anorexic child. I hope that after consulting this book you will be reassured. You can and should help and there are lots of things that you can do which will alter the course of the illness.

Although both boys and girls suffer from eating disorders, there are many more girls than boys among those affected. For simplicity, the feminine pronoun has been used in this book, but it should not be understood to exclude boys.

CHAPTER ONE

What is an eating disorder?

The eating disorders anorexia nervosa and bulimia nervosa are very different and separate illnesses although they both involve a distorted attitude to food.

Much of the information contained herein will be useful for the parents of sufferers of both illnesses. Throughout the book I have dealt with both illnesses together and pointed out the differences where appropriate.

THE HISTORY

Anorexia nervosa was referred to as early as three centuries ago, in 1669, by Dr John Reynolds in describing a girl who began to 'abstain from all solid food'. She seldom took more then 'the juice of a roasted raisin'. In 1694, Richard Moreton described a 16-year-old boy who had 'a total want of appetite'. This boy recovered when advised to 'abandon his studies, use riding and go into the country air'. The term anorexia nervosa was first used in 1873, when it was noted that there was no physical cause for the condition of those affected. An eminent French physician, Lasegue, published an article in which he wrote that the prognosis was good if the patient could be separated from her family.

Although the condition bulimia nervosa was described relatively recently in 1979, the word bulimia was used as early as the fourteenth century. Bulimia means 'ox hunger' and describes people who eat huge quantities of food. There are many examples dating back hundreds of years of people who overate and then vomited.

THE CAUSES

The causes of anorexia nervosa are complex and poorly understood. We know certain facts about anorexia which should give us some clues as to its causes. It is a disorder which mainly affects women and is rarely seen in Third World countries. We know that eating disorders are prevalent in groups such as models and dancers for whom thinness is very highly valued. We know that the incidence of eating disorders is increasing. We know that a person is three times more likely to develop an eating disorder if a close relative is affected. The fact that eating disorders run in families could be either because it is genetic or because those affected are living in the same family environment.

Studies done on identical and non-identical twins show that there is probably a genetic element to anorexia nervosa, suggesting that perhaps sufferers have a specific sort of personality. Studies of identical twins with anorexia show that in about 50 per cent of cases, both twins suffer from the illness. The percentage is a lot less for non-identical twins, pointing to a genetic component. Clearly environmental influences, especially the type of family in which she lives, must play an important part. There is great debate as to whether or not there is a biological cause for anorexia, whether or not we can measure abnormally high or abnormally low quantities of certain chemicals in the bodies of people who suffer from anorexia nervosa. But it seems likely that genetic, environmental and biological factors all work together and contribute to the causes of eating disorders.

ALL IN THE MIND?

Until 1930, doctors were still arguing as to whether anorexia nervosa was primarily a physiological problem or purely a psychological condition. Most doctors are now agreed that any physical symptoms are the effect rather than the cause of anorexia nervosa. The main features of anorexia nervosa are severe weight loss, loss of periods in girls and a relentless pursuit of thinness. The main feature of bulimia nervosa is the rapid consumption of huge quantities of food, so-called bingeing, followed by purging. The purging can take the form of self-induced vomiting or laxative abuse or both.

Some children who are anorexic would never dream of bingeing but if they are made to eat more food than they think is normal they might choose to make themselves vomit. These children are not suffering from bulimia nervosa but nevertheless the problems caused by their vomiting and the way you should handle it are essentially the same.

WHO IS AFFECTED?

Anorexia nervosa is a life-threatening condition affecting as many as one in a hundred schoolchildren. It affects both girls and boys but probably 10 times as many girls. There is some evidence to suggest that individuals may be born with a genetic predisposition to develop anorexia nervosa. An obsessive, perfectionist character may well be the predisposing characteristic. The average age of onset is 16 years, but this appears to be gradually dropping. We have treated a six-year-old girl who displayed the classic signs of anorexia nervosa. Some research suggests that the incidence of new cases could be doubling every decade. Six to 10 per cent of anorexic patients die as a direct result of their starvation or from suicide. This means that by far the largest percentage of patients with an eating disorder can be treated. You may find this hopeful statistic reassuring at times when progress with your child appears slow or nonexistent.

Twenty or 30 years ago, anorexia was confined mainly to middle-class white children. Now it attacks all groups of society regardless of social class or ethnic origins. The younger the age of onset the poorer the prognosis, and it is therefore vital that these youngsters are treated quickly and expertly.

It is extremely rare for children to develop bulimia nervosa but not so rare for anorexic children to vomit. Bulimia nervosa is something which more frequently begins in the late teens or early twenties but occasionally we see much younger teenagers who suffer from it. We certainly see far fewer patients who suffer from bulimia than anorexia at Rhodes Farm, but this may well be because most bulimic patients can be managed as out-patients and do not come into residential care. In the general population, however, there are probably 10 times as many bulimics as there are anorexics.

Like children suffering from anorexia, bulimics have a fear of gaining weight. Like anorexics, bulimics have a morbid fear of becoming fat and worry constantly about their weight. Many bulimics however have a normal or near normal weight and their illness goes undetected for many years. Teenagers who become bulimic have usually either been anorexic or have tried unsuccessfully to diet and see bulimia as an easier way to control their weight.

We have seen a huge increase in the number of people suffering from bulimia nervosa over the past 30 years. Some researchers who questioned women on their eating habits found that as many as 20 per cent of women may suffer from bulimia at some stage in their life.

WHY IS THE INCIDENCE OF EATING DISORDERS INCREASING?

Over the last few decades the average size of women has increased, thought to be due to better nutrition in childhood. Dress manufacturers have had to increase the measurement of all their standard sizes. On the other hand, fashion models and our idea of the perfect body have become increasingly thinner. It is becoming more and more difficult to bridge the gap between what is normal and what is considered beautiful. Cosmetics companies and diet firms lead us to believe that our bodies are made of clay. They tell us that by exercising and going on special diets anyone can make their body conform to whatever shape is fashionable. For most of us this is impossible, and even dedicated dieting does not bring contentment. The 'perfect' shape will still elude the majority. Not surprisingly, most teenagers are doomed to disappointment as they watch their bodies change into adulthood and realize that they are not destined to be 5′ 9″ and a size 10.

Although many teenagers will feel dissatisfied every time they turn the pages of a fashion magazine, most of them have enough self-confidence to accept their less than perfect bodies and continue with their life. However, increasing numbers of children are not even waiting for puberty to decide that nature needs a helping hand if they are ever to look like Julia Roberts. Evidence of a low self-esteem often precedes dieting and in many cases this need for self-improvement, to at least have a perfect body, triggers the rigorous diet. Those who choose to change their body shape often do so in the belief that being thin will bring confidence and popularity.

When a child first joins the other 50 per cent or so of their class who purport to be on a diet and actually lose weight, they are something of a phenomenon. Losing weight on a 'diet' is not something that most schoolchildren ever achieve and to succeed in this way attracts both praise and envy. For a child whose self-esteem is very low, suddenly to be able to attract such attention certainly reinforces their will to continue. Some will feel that they have at last found something they are good at, while others will have found something else they can succeed in which takes them one step nearer to the perfection they seek. Giving up the one thing in life that you really feel you are good at and are praised for isn't easy, and this obviously plays some part in the fact that these children don't stop dieting even when they are by far the thinnest children in their group.

Being thin is not the answer to problem relationships or a lack of self-confidence. We can all think of overweight, very successful people who are fun to be with and who have lots of friends. Equally there are many very thin people who are still unhappy about themselves and their lives and are very boring company. Most children, anorexic and potentially anorexic will freely admit that they do not choose their friends by the size of their thighs. They see that a lively personality and a caring attitude are what draws them to want to be friends with someone. Somehow, although they can see this is the case for them, they still believe that they will not have friends or be popular unless they achieve a size 8 dress size. The media has a lot to answer for. All too often we see classically anorexic girls who are called supermodels and are paid a vast sum of money to act as role models as well as clothes models to our impressionable youngsters.

Children who are just beginning to display worrying signs of overconcern about their weight and shape can often be helped to think more sensibly with help from parents and teachers. One can point out what an enormous variation there is amongst both children and adults when it comes to height, weight and body shape. There is a surprisingly small number of people who fit into the 'perfect' category of being very tall, slim and well proportioned. One can find fault with almost everyone one knows or sees in the street, each has an imperfection or two, but most manage nevertheless to find partners, careers and happiness.

A useful exercise is to examine critically one of the many mannequins displayed in fashion shop windows. Their height and shape are so grossly out of proportion that no one, not even the supermodels, could really be like that. Their legs are too long and their waists are so small that even size 10 dresses need great tucks of fabric to be pinned behind. The fashion industry is not selling reality, just an unachievable dream. Marilyn Monroe was a size 16 and still regarded by most as attractive. One wonders if this unerring drive towards waif-like bodies is driven by men or women. Certainly many of the Page Three girls are neatly positioned to disguise the fat that is inevitably deposited on their hips and tummies as well as their breasts; very few of them could claim to be a size 10.

At a time when a child's body is growing and changing rapidly as well as their body image, (i.e the mental image they are forming of the shape of their body and the way they look) a parent must be aware of these potentially damaging external influences and work to counter them. Puberty is a difficult time for many children. The responsibilities of adulthood loom and they may feel ill equipped to deal with them. It is a time when children change schools, and often find themselves alone in a strange environment before they make new friends. As their starvation continues, victims become depressed and even more self-critical. They often have such strong feelings of worthlessness that they believe dieting can be the only thing they are good at.

DIETING

Dieting has become a national pastime in this country. Ninety per cent of women diet at some time in their life. Although the number of men on diets is increasing, it is nowhere near the same level. If one does a survey amongst women, half of them are dieting at any one time. Even children as young as eight talk of their need to diet. There are more and more diet products on the market and yet the number of overweight people is increasing.

In 1987, 12 per cent of women were overweight and in 1991 it had risen to 16 per cent, with the percentage of overweight men also rising from 8 to 12 per cent over the same period. Despite the number of people on diets, very few people ever succeed in losing weight and staying slim. Research shows that the majority of people who lose weight by following very low calorie diets, i.e. fewer than 800 kcal a day, regain their lost weight very quickly when they cease to diet. There is evidence to show that people who diet frequently actually gain more weight than people who do not diet at all. They deprive themselves of food and are then prone to bingeing.

When a dieter consumes more than the amount of food that they have set for themselves, i.e. breaks their diet, they go on to eat far more food than people not on a diet. People not on diets compensate for a large intake of high calorific food by automatically restricting their intake for a while following their large meal. Dieters do the opposite and as a consequence often put on more weight than they lose by dieting.

We are also seeing an increase in the number of overweight children in this country. Research seems to indicate that it is due to a huge reduction in the amount of exercise that children now take compared to 20 years ago. It does not seem to be related to an increased intake of 'junk' food as was once thought. Children used to walk to school, come home and play football or games in the street. Nowadays they are driven to school and play video games. If your child does have a weight problem, encouraging her to do more exercise or to join a sports club can be a very useful way of helping her control her weight.

Why is it that we all set such store by being thin? Why is it that so many children feel so unhappy about the shape of their body that they either diet or worry about it, or both? A recent survey carried out in schools shows that 57 per cent of the girls and 17 per cent of the boys claimed to be dieting. With only 4 per cent of schoolchildren overweight it is hardly surprising that eating disorders are increasing so dramatically.

At some stage most children announce their intention to diet. In the majority of cases you will not see any evidence of a reduction in their intake of food or any noticeable weight loss. If your child does lose weight you should be wary. You should begin by weighing and measuring her to see if indeed she is overweight. Up to 105 per cent weight-for-height ratio is a perfectly good weight. (See charts on pp172-7)

But even overweight children should not be encouraged to diet drastically. Most of them are eating more calories per day than they need to maintain growth and daily life. If they can be encouraged simply to cut down to a level which is normal so that they no longer gain weight, then natural growth will slim them down without them actually having to lose weight. And many children who think they are overweight are in fact within the normal range.

IF YOUR CHILD IS OVERWEIGHT

If your child is 2 – 3kg overweight you can help her cut down her food intake by just 250 calories a day, which might mean simply stopping her eating sweets and biscuits between meals. A small cut in intake like this will probably allow you to keep her weight stable. As children put on weight every year as part of their normal growth and development, she can slim down simply by not gaining any weight for a period of time.

This can be achieved more easily than trying to lose weight. If your child does in fact need to lose weight, you can help her achieve this without making her anxious and concerned about food. As parents, you control her pocket money and prepare her meals and snacks so it should be relatively easy to adjust her food intake so that she loses weight very gradually. You will need to get some idea of what she eats for lunch at school and adjust her evening meal accordingly. This could be a salad if she tells you she has eaten fish and chips, or something a bit more substantial if she has eaten a salad for lunch.

Counting calories is a very sure way of regulating her intake but do make sure that she is not party to your calculations – you do not want to make her obsessed with food. She will be able to lose ½kg a week if you reduce her intake by 500 calories a day. You should be able to do this safely without her feeling deprived or becoming preoccupied with food. Weigh her twice a week to make sure that her weight loss is not excessive. There again, be careful not to have lengthy discussions with her about her weight. Try to weigh her without her seeing the display.

Dieting in most people does not lead to an eating disorder. Many children experiment with dieting but only a small percentage actually become ill. When it comes to dieting, anorexic children and potential anorexics have a will power which guarantees them success. Perfection is their key word and unlike the majority of us who diet every Monday morning until lunchtime, or until offered our first chocolate bar, they do not deviate from their goal. One-third of anorexic children have been among the 4 per cent of children in this country who are overweight. They will often recount a joke or cruel comment which triggered their determination to lose weight.

DIETING MYTHS

There is a vast array of conflicting and often downright wrong advice on dieting available, much of it specifically targeted at teenagers. Despite the promise of tighter controls on the advertising of diet foods there are still many so-called diet products available whose claims to aid weight loss are at best dubious. Magazines are also full of articles about weight and dieting, many of these directed at teenagers. Often these not only encourage them to follow very low-calorie regimes, they also make false claims about the effects of their diets. The nutritional advice given is often completely contrary to that which would be given by a doctor or a qualified nutritionist.

There is also an endless stream of diets and exercise videos aimed at spot-reducing a particular part of the body. Children and many adults often follow useless advice in the hope of reducing their thighs or tummy. The distribution of body fat is something which is genetically determined. Women have between 20 per cent and 28 per cent body fat and men have between 12 per cent and 16 per cent. Some very slim individuals appear to store their body fat reserves internally, surrounding the intestine and kidneys. Others distribute their fat evenly, and some carry the majority of their fat on a certain area of the body. This may be buttocks, breasts, tummy, thighs, etc. If one looks at a person's natural body shape, it is very often similar to that of their parents and grandparents. By dieting we can lose fat from our fat stores but what we cannot do is determine from where that fat will be lost. If someone who is pear-shaped diets, there is a probability that she will lose yet more weight from her already normal upper body before any fat is lost from her thighs. No amount of waving our legs in the air or other exercises will encourage fat loss from a particular part of our body. We occasionally see girls who have begun dieting because they felt that their legs were too fat. Three stone later they still believe that their legs are too fat, certainly they are still not in proportion to the rest of her body, and they could well die before they ever achieve a body shape that they are happy with.

Exercise is a useful way for overweight people to burn off excess calories and it also helps speed metabolism so that one burns off more calories in the course of a normal day. Exercise in moderation is a useful way for normal-weight people to keep fit, or for overweight people to speed their metabolism, but it will never help reduce the size of thighs or tummy other than by helping overall weight loss.

One of the most important things you can do for your child in the way of prevention is to arm yourself with solid nutritional facts about a healthy diet. This is not as simple as it sounds faced as you will be with a plethora of conflicting advice. Arguments rage between doctors and nutritionists about what we should and should not eat. You will need to be able to dispel some of the myths of healthy eating and to understand the basics of a normal teenage diet. (See Chapter 6 – Living with an anorexic child)

GOOD AND BAD FOOD

There is no such thing as healthy food or unhealthy food, there are only healthy and unhealthy diets. Fruit, which is generally regarded as healthy, becomes very unhealthy as most anorexics learn to their peril when eaten to the exclusion of other foods. No one should be encouraged to live on chocolate or chips but taken as part of a balanced diet they are excellent foods. Parents should see that their children eat plenty of fresh fruit and vegetables, cereals and protein in the form of fish and meat every day. Once they have eaten these vital foods, they can happily consume any extra calories they require in the form of chips, crisps or chocolate. Very few children overeat and in most cases only eat when they are hungry.

Among the children referred to us, we see more than our fair share with parents, mothers in particular, who are what I would describe as fitness fanatics. They often stick rigidly to a low-fat diet, have never allowed their children to eat crisps, sweets or chocolate and regularly attend aerobics classes, often taking their children with them. Low-fat diets should be reserved for overweight people trying to lose weight. Children and adults need 30–32 per cent fat in their daily allowance. As a nation we have become obsessed with low-fat diets, an obsession fuelled by government publications urging us to eat certain quantities of certain foods and suggesting we involve children as young as seven in this anxiety-provoking exercise. There is very little evidence to suggest that what children eat has any bearing whatsoever on their incidence of heart disease in later life. Instead research seems to indicate that before the age of 25 our diet has very little effect on the incidence of heart disease. What is more, we know that women are protected by their hormones until menopause and lay down little or no fat in their arteries until this time. Thus there is every reason to suggest that we should be telling our children to stop worrying about what they eat, eat a normal varied diet and assure them that no harm will come to them.

Children should be allowed to snack on the normal foods that children like as long as they are eating three balanced and nutritious meals a day. Children typically take only about half their daily calorific intake during their three meals, the rest is taken in the way of snacks. This 'grazing' is very normal and there is no need to discourage it unless one finds that snacks are making up so much of their diet that they are not hungry at meal-times and therefore do not eat the protein which these meals should provide. During their growth spurt, children often eat more than 4,000 kcals a day. They need to snack regularly on high-calorie foods if they are not to become hungry. Most children regulate their eating well, and it is unusual for children to eat when they are not hungry.

It is important not to discourage children from eating by telling them that they will get fat. Very few children are fat so it is unlikely to happen. If a child eats a high-calorie meal she will compensate automatically by cutting down her intake later in the day. Children need high-energy foods that will sustain them through what will be a very active afternoon. So, along with the carrots or celery that you put in their school lunch boxes, you must ensure that they get adequate carbohydrates. They are not on diets. I have heard many teachers complaining about how tired their charges are in the afternoon. They often blame it on late bedtimes but I am convinced that low-fat, low-calorie lunches are more to blame for their lethargy. We should try to relieve children of the idea of good and bad foods, and try to prevent the guilt felt by adults rubbing off onto our children. Food is a very important social focus for most of us; it is sad if we cannot allow our children to enjoy it.

CHAPTER TWO

The signs: what to look out for

When I first noticed that Sandra wasn't eating I thought it was just a passing phase. I didn't think my child would develop anorexia, she had always loved her food. When I began to coax her and became aware of the resistance, I really panicked. I felt completely impotent. A mother's role is to feed her children and mine was steadfastly refusing my most tempting meals. My GP seemed to think I was a neurotic mother and didn't share my anxieties at all. I felt very alone and didn't know where to turn.

She was showing all the symptoms I had read about anorexia but I still couldn't persuade anyone to take my worries seriously. I wasn't until she began to look gaunt and fainted one morning that my doctor and family took notice. I felt guilty that I hadn't made more of a fuss and blamed myself for her illness. I was sure it was my fault that she was refusing food, it had to be something I had done. As she continued to lose weight despite seeing dieticians and psychiatrists, I was sure that she would die and that no one would be able to help. There is so little help for these children and even less help for their parents.

WHAT TO LOOK OUT FOR IN ANOREXIA

One of the first things you might notice is that your child has lost a lot of weight or seems much thinner than usual. Apart from this general awareness, you can look out for these specific signs:

1. Preoccupation with weight

The most common symptom of the illness is a preoccupation with being extremely thin and a terrible dread of becoming fat. Children with anorexia often jump on and off the scales 20 times a day to make sure they are not putting on weight. They constantly compare their bodies to those of friends and convince themselves that most people are thinner than they are.

2. Concern with 'healthy' diet – cutting calories

Of course the one characteristic of every case of anorexia is that of weight loss. One of the principal features in the diagnosis of anorexia nervosa is the loss of 20 per cent or more of a normal body weight. The illness often begins with what appears to be a normal diet or by the child saying that she wants to eat more healthily. Understanding that fat has more calories than any other type of food, anorexic children cut fat out of their diet very early on in their illness. They often justify it on the grounds of healthy eating and trying to keep a healthy heart. They may begin by cutting out sweets and chocolate. They then graduate to not drinking milk or eating butter, cheese or other foods containing fat. At some stage in the process they usually become vegetarian and thus they have an excuse for not eating meat and cutting out a few more calories.

As well as cutting down on food, some anorexics restrict their intake of fluids. They realize quickly that a dehydrated body weighs less than a hydrated one and thus in the late stages of the illness when weight loss becomes more difficult, they may resort to not drinking.

LARA'S STORY

Lara became obsessed with food when she was about 12 years old. She was shown a film at school about slaughtering animals and immediately decided to become vegetarian. Within a few months she began to buy calorie books and became obsessed with counting calories and avoiding fat. She followed me into the kitchen and watched me cook. She complained when I used oil to fry things and hated to see me put cream in any of the sauces. She loved to cook and made enormous cakes for the family, usually covered in cream and chocolate. She pushed us all into eating huge chunks of these cakes but never made any attempt to eat them herself.

She examined the calorie content of every packet in the kitchen and consulted the nutrition information on every yoghurt pot. In a matter of months she was eating only plain boiled vegetables and a little fruit. As well as not eating, she was exercising endlessly. She never sat down, she walked the dog, she emptied the dishwasher, she cleaned the cupboards and found endless excuses to go up and down the stairs. She would not go to the cinema or the theatre because she couldn't bear to sit still for that length of time. When we stopped her going on endless walks and bike rides and forbade her to go swimming, we then caught her exercising endlessly in her room.

Her weight loss was dramatic and within a few weeks she was so weak she was no longer able to exercise. She looked emaciated, her eyes were sunken, her teeth seemed to protrude because she had lost even the fat from her face. Her arms and legs were like sticks and her hip bones protruded. Despite her skeletal appearance she constantly asked for reassurance that she was not fat, and gazed at herself in the mirror for long periods of time.

She refused to go to the doctor so we asked for a home visit from a psychiatrist. He insisted that she was immediately admitted to an eating disorders unit. She was by now extremely emaciated and had no strength at all. Nevertheless, she tried to resist this move to send her to a unit where she would have to eat. She promised us that if we left her at home for one more week she would show us that she was in fact able to eat and get better and did not need to be admitted to a unit. I am ashamed to say that we fell for this and another week went by when rather than the gaining weight she lost even more. At the end of that week despite her protests we drove her to the clinic.

Once in the clinic she seemed to co-operate with the programme – she certainly ate what was put in front of her. We later learnt that she hid a lot of the food, that she vomited and also exercised endlessly in the toilet or bathroom when she was left alone. When the staff realized that she was not gaining weight, they began to supervise her more closely and this produced the weight gain they were expecting. For the following month she continued to try and beat the system. Whenever she was left alone, she found ways to cheat and avoid putting on weight. She refused to speak to her therapist and contributed *nothing at all in family therapy sessions. She ended up spending most of her time being supervised by a nurse.*

As her weight increased she became more rational, more positive and began to take responsibility for herself. She did however continue to tell us that as soon as she left the unit she intended to lose all the weight again. This upset us greatly but after a while we realized that this was exactly what she intended. She often said things that she knew would hurt us. It was clear that she was angry and resentful because we had forced her to accept treatment. As we were her nearest and dearest she chose to blame us. There were times when we despaired and could not imagine that she would ever recover. We stuck with the programme despite her pleading and begging to be allowed home. Just before her discharge we made it quite clear to her that if she lost even 1kg at home we would see that outings, trips, activities and if necessary school would be stopped until she restored her weight.

We had a few minor battles when she returned home but once she realized that we meant what we said and that we had no intention of allowing her to lose even 1kg, she was able to relax in the knowledge that it was no longer her decision. Two years on she is now a happy, lively girl, still slim, still worried about what she eats but leading a normal life.

3. Rituals

A ritualistic way of eating is strangely common to many anorexics. It involves putting very small amounts on the fork, maybe even eating peas and baked beans one at a time. If fish or chicken is prepared in breadcrumbs, they are often picked off, even if the child intends to eat them later. Apples are cut into tiny pieces with a knife, each tiny piece eaten individually or dropped into a yoghurt. Food is often mashed and spread over a large area of the plate, this is presumably so that as much can be left on the plate as possible. Nuts are often picked out of muesli due to their high calorific value. Anorexics often put water on their cereals and eat dry bread and they often consume gallons of diet fizzy drinks. They eat vast quantities of fruit and vegetables which have few or no calories. Although the rituals are most commonly to do with the way food is prepared and eaten it can involve other tasks such as exercise routines. We will come onto this a little later.

Eating the same thing every day is another hallmark of anorexia nervosa. Eating the same small bowl of cereal for breakfast, the same piece of fruit for lunch and exactly the same evening meal is very common. They feel safe eating in this routine way and can be sure that they will not suddenly put on weight. They are so afraid that if they add a few more calories than usual they will gain several kilos overnight. Obviously this unvaried diet is unhealthy, both physically and psychologically and must not be allowed to become a habit.

4. Hiding food

Many anorexic children choose to eat alone or in their rooms so that they can hide or dispose of food, or simply not to arouse suspicion about how little they are eating. Some sufferers don't like to eat in front of people because they feel greedy and think that they are so fat that they shouldn't be eating at all. Many children hide food in their rooms in places where it will be found very easily, which is probably a cry for help.

5. Exercise

In an effort to lose weight more quickly some anorexics turn to exercise. This can be surreptitious, constantly finding excuses to run upstairs, walk the dog until he begs for mercy, or more overt, cycling, swimming and aerobics with a few hundred sit-ups thrown in for good measure.

Many children mistakenly believe that they will burn off more calories by standing up than they will by sitting. It is not unusual to see these children standing up watching the television, writing letters or doing their homework. They feel guilty when they sit down and, even when forced to do so, sit on the edge of their seat with their muscles tensed or continuing to exercise their legs and feet under the table. They are often reluctant to go to bed, walking around their rooms until the small hours and then setting their alarm clock in order to get up early. As they become weaker they often have to abandon exercise and resort to cutting down still further on their food intake. As the illness progresses, the need to concentrate resolutely on food and calories takes over completely and even exams and schoolwork are abandoned.

A habit common to anorexic children is sleeping with the window wide open, having very little in the way of bed covers and walking around in the depth of winter in shorts and a T-shirt. This bizarre behaviour is aimed at burning more calories in making the body work harder to keep warm. Yet again, the few calories that are consumed in this way cannot be worth the discomfort which must be endured.

6. Your child may become depressed and antisocial

At some stage in their illness most children become withdrawn and antisocial. There are two reasons for this behaviour. The first is to do with low self-esteem and feelings of worthlessness, which often accompany anorexia. The second is purely to do with the effects of starvation, which causes depression and lethargy. Initially they may withdraw from their friends simply because most teenage activities involve grabbing a pizza or a hamburger and they want to avoid situations where they may be pressured into eating.

Thoughts of weight, food and exercise fill every waking hour and understandably these children have little time left to think about enjoying themselves. Most of the children we see have forgotten how it feels to be a carefree child who laughs, jokes and generally loves people and life. All the *joie de vivre* has long gone from their lives and they exist rather than live. Their relentless pursuit of thinness leaves no room for thoughts of others and they often become selfish while superficially retaining a pretence of caring.

7. Missed periods

Lack of periods is an early but nevertheless serious sign that dieting has become out of control. It should be taken as proof that a child needs urgent medical help and is a situation which cannot be allowed to continue.

8. Obsessive-compulsive behaviour

Your child may exhibit signs of obsessive-compulsive behaviour.

This can take many forms such as, for example, extreme cleanliness, excessive handwashing or worries about germs in general. Some children wash their hands so often that they become red and sore. Obsessive tidiness is another common feature, bedrooms, cupboards and drawers being arranged in impeccable order.

Perfectionism is another common characteristic of anorexic children. The majority of children who suffer from anorexia nervosa are high academic achievers. They want to produce perfect pieces of schoolwork, often spending hours on their homework and then tearing up page after page because it's not perfect. This striving for perfection leads them to work extremely hard. They are bitterly disappointed if they achieve anything below an 'A' grade.

9. Clothes

Anorexic children tend to dress in a similar way. Quite frequently they wear many layers of clothing in an attempt to keep warm. They wear dowdy, scruffy loose clothes, usually trousers or long skirts.

Whether this baggy clothing is to disguise their so-called fatness as they claim, or whether it is an attempt to cover what they really know is a very thin body I have yet to discover but the anorexic 'uniform' is unmistakable. While some anorexic children are obsessively fastidious about personal hygiene, others do not wash regularly and wear the same clothes day after day so that they cannot be washed. This behaviour seems to go along with their lack of self-esteem, as often these children quite openly say that they do not like themselves. Wearing dull old clothes with holes in reflects how they feel about themselves. Another common reason for wearing the same garments is that one particular waistband acts as reassuring proof that they are not gaining weight. Washing garments often slightly shrinks them and panics anorexic children into believing they are getting fatter.

As the illness advances, the sufferers have problems keeping up their body temperatures and huddle close to radiators and often burn themselves on hot water bottles. At this stage, they will not feel well enough to have fun with friends.

ANN'S STORY

Ann was 13 when I first noticed that she was getting thinner. She had always been a plump child and at first I was pleased that she was losing some weight. It seemed as though there were only a few weeks between me thinking how good she looked and suddenly panicking because she looked gaunt and ill.

She continued to lose weight even though she seemed to be eating very well. She sat down with us every night and ate a large plate of food. She had become vegetarian just before she started to lose weight and always prepared her own food. It wasn't until I recounted the history to a doctor that I realized how strange it was that my 13-year-old was cooking her own food. It was the same doctor who told me how few calories there were in the vegetables and pasta she had been eating. Ann continued to lose weight – she wouldn't eat for me at all. We rowed constantly about her food. My husband and I rowed too about how we should handle her. He wanted to be really tough with her while I thought that we shouldn't push her too much. I rather she ate a little than nothing at all.

WHAT TO LOOK OUT FOR IN BULIMIA

1. Bingeing

The first thing you might notice if your child is bulimic is that vast quantities of food are disappearing. Packets of biscuits, cakes, puddings and sweets are favourites. Some sufferers do not risk taking food from the cupboards where its loss may be noticed but spend large quantities of money on buying their own. If this is the case you might instead look out for lots of empty packets. They are very likely to deny that they have eaten so much food and try to blame its disappearance on others.

2. Vomiting

If your child is vomiting, you will see her disappear to the bathroom or to her bedroom very soon after finishing her meal. The easiest time to vomit is just after having eaten. Standing outside the bathroom door is a fruitless occupation as children who vomit learn to do so very quietly and quickly. You are unlikely to hear very much. What you will notice and which is much harder to disguise is the characteristic smell. This smell hangs around in the bathroom for some time and the children themselves very often smell of vomit.

Although many children who vomit do not want to be discovered, some do want people to know. It is not unusual for bulimic children to vomit into polythene bags and leave them in the bedroom in places where they will be found. This is a real cry for help and should not be ignored. A large percentage of people who suffer from bulimia are depressed. Some researchers think that bulimia is in fact a depressive illness but others think that the bulimia comes first and the depression follows from it. Even the sufferers who are not clinically depressed are usually extremely unhappy. They feel very bad about themselves to the point of self-loathing. After bingeing bulimics often feel very anxious, and giving in to the vomiting often relieves their anxiety and makes them feel better.

Another sign to look out for is redness or even calluses on the knuckles of the second and third fingers. People who induce vomiting often put their fingers into their throat and their teeth catch on their knuckles as they retch. When this is done repeatedly, it leaves an almost permanent mark on the hands, a real tell-tale sign. Occasionally, the children retch so much that the repeated strain bursts blood vessels in their eyes and they end up with extremely red eyes.

Other than being aware that she disappears quickly from the table after meals, there are very few ways of spotting vomiting and this is why it is so dangerous. We hear of cases where teenagers have vomited for many years before seeking help and no one in their family has ever suspected.

3. Exercise

Many bulimics over-exercise in the same way as anorexics do in an attempt to control their weight and to compensate for the food they have eaten.

EFFECTS OF VOMITING

There are many other ill effects which are not immediately noticeable to a parent but of which the sufferers will be aware. Very often the retching causes slight bleeding and it is not unusual for bulimics to see some blood mixed with their vomit. Sometimes this bleeding can be much more serious. It can be caused by the retching being so severe that it tears a blood vessel and could cause fatal bleeding. This can happen even after a relatively short history of vomiting.

Another cause of bleeding is ulceration. Unlike the stomach, the gullet or oesophagus is not designed to withstand attack by acids. When the stomach contents are regularly regurgitated through the gullet, the acid can cause serious damage to the lining, which then results in ulceration and bleeding.

People who vomit develop puffy faces, the salivary glands just behind the cheeks swell and enlarge, giving the sufferer a hamster-like appearance. Knowing that this is likely to occur with chronic vomiting sometimes does worry children enough to make them stop. Doing something that makes them look particularly unattractive certainly defeats the object of vomiting, which is presumably to make them look more attractive.

Persistent vomiting can lower potassium levels to a dangerous degree. As well as upsetting the heart rhythm, this can cause swollen ankles and legs, and is a very common problem in people who vomit persistently. It is a worrying sign that something is amiss.

The teeth become damaged quite early on when people vomit as the acid attacks them as it does the eosophagus. The enamel is softened and then eroded by the constant exposure to acid. Long-term vomiters lose all their teeth to decay. Some children think that if they clean their teeth very well after vomiting that they will protect them, but this is not the case. After vomiting, the enamel on the teeth is so soft that brushing damages it even more, it certainly does not prevent damage.

About 50 per cent of people who vomit do not have periods, or if they do, they are very irregular. This is thought to be due to the fluctuation in their weight and their poor diet. One of the long-term consequences of vomiting is the development of a condition called polycystic ovaries. The ovaries develop many cysts over their surface, which results in impaired fertility.

LAXATIVES

Some bulimics induce vomiting after a binge and then take large quantities of laxatives. They think that by doing so they will be getting rid of some of the food they have eaten.

Research suggests that many schoolchildren abuse laxatives in the hope of losing weight. Many anorexic children take laxatives, some because anorexia genuinely causes constipation and many more in the mistaken belief that laxatives prevent the absorption of calories. Amongst children with bulimia nervosa, laxative abuse is also very common. Laxatives have a great number of harmful side-effects. Most certainly they do not have any effect on the absorption of food. Every last calorie is extracted from the food long before the laxatives have any effect. Laxatives do nothing more than allow the normal waste from the body to be passed out with lots of water rather than dry as happens in constipation. The waste is exactly the same with or without laxatives, it does not contain a single calorie. Passing out abnormal quantities of water with the stools does however cause dehydration, which in turn makes the body weigh less. Each litre of water passed out of the body makes the body weight 1kg less. When people who jump on and off the scales several times a day take laxatives, they will see a weight loss and will thus convince themselves that laxatives help them lose weight. What many children do not realize is that as soon as they drink a glass or two of water, the water balance will be corrected and their weight will rise again. As well as causing severe dehydration, which can cause kidney stones, laxatives can irritate the bowel and cause bleeding. Prolonged use of laxatives can cause permanent damage to the gut so that it will never again function normally. Laxative abuse also causes the body's potassium balance to be disturbed and brings with it the risk of a heart attack or death.

Children should be told what a waste of time it is to take laxatives. They risk serious damage to their health without a single calorie being saved.

SIGNS THAT YOUR CHILD NEEDS URGENT MEDICAL CARE

Sometimes despite everyone's best efforts there comes a time when a decision has to be made to admit a patient to hospital.

If you are unable to help your child eat at home and her weight falls 20 per cent below a normal weight for her age and height (see pp172-7), she needs to be admitted to hospital. If your daughter is vomiting on a regular basis, whatever her weight, you need to admit her.

There are several other dangerous signs, which can be picked up on physical examination, that also require immediate hospital treatment. These would be signs of dehydration caused by a refusal to drink or because of vomiting or laxative abuse. Symptoms of a poor circulation such as a low blood pressure or a slow pulse would also need urgent treatment. Another reason for admitting an anorexic child regardless of her weight would be if she were severely depressed.

There are several reasons why a bulimic might need in-patient treatment. One reason would be if her vomiting was so severe that she was losing weight and her weight had fallen below a safe level. Other reasons to admit would be if the persistent vomiting had caused a dangerous drop in her potassium levels, or if the child were so depressed that she felt suicidal.

As with anorexic patients, it is unlikely that your child will be volunteering to go into hospital. It is more likely that she is denying vomiting, doesn't think she has a problem, and doesn't know what all the fuss is about. You must take the advice of the professionals and do what is right, not what your ill child wants.

CHAPTER THREE

What to do if you suspect your child has an eating disorder

If you have not been in the habit of making rules and sticking to them, you need to sit down with your child and explain that you feel your laxity in the past has not been helpful and that from now on things are going to change. Having explained that there will now be swift and immediate sanctions with no second chance, you must carry out your threats immediately if the rules are broken.

FIRST STEPS WITH SUSPECTED ANOREXIA

If you suspect that your child is not eating properly you need to see what is actually happening to her weight. Some children eat very little at meal-times, either because they intend to diet or because they crave attention. After the meal when no one is looking, they eat the leftovers or raid the fridge. These children do not have an eating disorder and they do not lose weight.

Weigh your child for three consecutive weeks so that you can see exactly the situation as regards her weight. If her weight is falling, alarm bells should ring. From birth until the age of 15 or 16, a child's weight should steadily increase every month. It certainly should not go backwards. You will find advice on what to do if your child needs to lose weight in Chapter One.

If she has only just started to diet and has not lost very much weight, you may well be able to nip this in the bud by being extremely firm.

Tell her she is to be weighed every week and explain that if she doesn't at least stabilise her weight, you will have to take her to see her GP. Make sure that you sit down with her to eat breakfast and an evening meal and give her a snack when she comes home from school. At the weekends you can see that she eats lunch as well. Serve her sensible size portions of normal food; don't be persuaded to prepare salads and low-calorie meals. Insist that she finishes what you give her. If she has not at least maintained her weight when you weigh her at the end of the week, you must increase her intake the week after.

If despite being very firm and vigilant she still loses weight you must consult your GP and ask to be referred to a child psychiatrist. In some cases you may not notice her cutting down on her food intake. This may be because you don't eat together very often or because she is very good at fooling you. There are several ways that anorexic children can appear to eat but still lose weight. If the first thing you notice is that she has become very thin or that her periods have stopped, you should go to your GP immediately.

If your child is pre-pubertal, be wary if her weight stays stable for any length of time. Her weight should be increasing and if she stays at the same weight for six months or a year, this will have the effect of her losing weight. Her peers will certainly have gained weight during the same time period.

Your GP might try for two or three weeks to help you encourage your child to eat and gain weight. He/she will be able to weigh her accurately, explain to her the consequences of not eating and talk to her about any problems she may have. If you are not able to help her gain a minimum of ½kg each week with the help of your GP then the next step is to be referred to a consultant child psychiatrist, who can arrange individual and family therapy and at the same time should be able to arrange for you to see a dietician. He/she should be able to give you some clear-cut advice on preparing high-calorie meals, which have a high fat content. Your child should continue to see your GP or a paediatrician on a weekly basis to have her weight, pulse and blood pressure monitored. She should also be seeing a therapist and attending family therapy with you. The extreme importance of therapy will be discussed later in this chapter.

For now it is sufficient to say that you must insist that your child sees her therapist each week and that you and your wife/husband or partner are free to attend family therapy meetings as required. Family therapy is probably the single most important component of any treatment programme aimed at helping children with eating disorders.

FIRST STEPS WITH SUSPECTED BULIMIA

First of all you should sit down with your child and tell her that you think she is vomiting. She may admit it and be pleased that someone has at last found out and confronted her problem. Whether she freely admits it or whether she denies it vehemently, the next step is the same. You must tell her about the long- and short-term consequences of vomiting. Be straight forward and don't beat about the bush – you are trying to frighten her so much that she will stop.

Having told her about the dangers, try to find out if there is anything particular that is worrying her. You are unlikely to find out one specific problem, she may deny that anything is wrong and simply tell you that she feels fat or is worried about getting fat. She might feel that everything is wrong and that her life is in turmoil. Whether or not you succeed in gaining some insight into what is driving her to feel so bad about herself, you will have to insist that she goes to see someone with whom she can talk. Your GP should be your first port of call. If you think that despite organising her a counsellor or therapist and making her aware of the risks she is taking she is still vomiting then you need to supervise her very closely.

Family therapy

Most clinicians treating young children suffering from bulimia nervosa would agree that family therapy has an important part to play in treating the illness. If you are asked to attend family therapy sessions, it is important that you go with an open mind and that you go as a family prepared to speak frankly about the problems there are within your family group. All families have problems. What differentiates families is the way they handle and confront their problems.

There are many theories about why it is that teenagers become bulimic and many of them involve the family. It is often thought that some children see bulimia as a way of getting attention or as a way of rebelling in a family where the more open rebellion commonly seen among teenage children is not an option. In these cases, family therapy can be extremely useful in helping the family identify problem areas and think about how it can nurture the child so that she no longer needs her bulimia.

Bulimic children may see their illness as a way of taking pressure off their parents' ailing marriage, or distracting a distressed mother. Again, these are issues which can be dealt with in family therapy and will not easily be resolved if the patient only receives individual therapy. Many families are reluctant to take part in family therapy and will try to justify their view that it will not help. They will say that there are no problems within their family, that everything is perfect and no help is needed. They will also explain that the child's siblings have been exposed to exactly the same environment and are fit and well.

This is proof that we cannot 'blame' the family for their children's illness, but it doesn't mean that the family could not change in some way so as to make their bulimic child better able to live within that family. The problem may be with the child who, for example, is unlike her siblings in being non-assertive and therefore needs help in getting her voice heard or worries recognized.

Through family therapy parents can be helped to see that

they have no need to feel guilty about their daughter's eating disorder. Parents of children with eating disorders often feel responsible or to blame for the child's condition, even though there is no evidence at all that families are the cause of eating problems. They often think that they are bad parents or that any marital problems have contributed to her illness. Through family therapy it should be possible to help parents understand the illness and to dispel any guilt they may feel. They should be encouraged and supported in their struggle against her illness. The parents are very important allies, both to the sufferer and to the professionals trying to help her. Parents are ideally placed to help deal with the symptoms of the illness, i.e. bingeing, vomiting and exercising, and also to help the therapist by highlighting relevant issues.

SEEKING HELP
More on family therapy

Research has shown us that family therapy is a very important part of treating young children who have not had their eating disorder for longer than three years. At Rhodes Farm we are so convinced of its necessity that we will not admit a child whose parents do not agree to attend together every two weeks for family therapy sessions. We also like to see the siblings and other important family members like partners or grandparents who might play a large part in the child's life. We don't always insist that everyone attends every meeting but that the two parents attend with their child, if both are present in her life, is vital. Many families feel threatened by very idea of family therapy. They think that we are somehow blaming the family for the difficulties and assuming them to be the cause of the problems. This is far from the case. Of course there are often problems in relationships between family members and very often it is helpful for the patient to be able to discuss these problems and try to find a solution to them. Sometimes it is simply a matter of the family finding a way of helping their child get better. This often involves changing the way members of the family function together. We always find that when we can see a change in the family dynamics we have a greater chance of seeing the patient recover. We sometimes see families in the situation we describe as 'stuck'. We either identify problems which no one is very motivated to deal with or the family denies the existence of problems and tells us everything is perfect. When this happens, we know we will be sending the child home to exactly the same worries that she had before, and with that a very high risk of relapse.

People are often puzzled by family therapy meetings and are unsure what is unexpected of them or what they are supposed to do. The therapist is there to facilitate the family in thinking about and solving any problems there may be. She is not there to ask lots of questions or tease out problems, more to encourage the family to identify things which might need discussion and resolution.

For this reason, family therapy sessions often begin by a few minutes of total silence. The family sometimes thinks that the therapist should be asking them pointed questions wheras in fact the therapist is waiting for the family to tell her what they would like to talk about during the session. It is important to be open and honest and not to hide things from the therapist.

Family secrets are not helpful when trying to work with the family.

Although it is easy to blame yourself for the problems your child may have, you must remember that no one is trying to apportion blame. Feelings of helplessness and guilt are common to families of anorexic children and you are not alone if you have these thoughts.

One of the important functions of family therapy is to unite the family in their task of feeding and nurturing their child. Once they can work together to do this, they begin to feel a little more positive and less helpless. If your child is to recover it is vital that you are in control, not your daughter. Family therapy sessions can be very emotional. Sometimes people say things which are hurtful. Sometimes the child becomes angry because the parents are trying to take charge. She has been in control for so long that she will not relinquish it easily. If she isn't getting her own way she might shout or be abusive, or she might run out of the session altogether. If she does this you will have to decide whether or not to go and bring her back and if so, who is the best person to do so.

The expression of anger and resentment in children who are undergoing treatment for an eating disorder is common. It often happens when they begin to eat and gain weight. For parents who are used to a child who has always been 'perfect' and has never confronted them, this can be a worrying change of personality. In fact, it is a very healthy sign and the child should be encouraged to express her emotions and share her anger. Anorexia nervosa is often seen as an illness where anger and pent up emotions are turned inwardly and suppressed.

Instead of telling people about their worries and anger as most teenagers do, they say nothing and take their anger out on their eating. It is an excellent sign when these children can express themselves verbally instead of having to starve themselves. This phase does not continue. Although one hopes the child will continue to be able to verbalise her feelings, her behaviour will not be quite so confrontational. Forewarned is forearmed so be aware that this phase is a normal part of the recovery process. The families of children with anorexia nervosa are described as people who have difficulty in expressing their emotions and also of confronting problems. When these children do become confrontational, they are therefore being extremely brave in moving away from the family's normal behaviour.

It is important to see family therapy as necessary because it is the family who can best deal with and control the symptoms of the child's disordered eating, not because the family is the cause of them. In some units family therapy sessions are conducted in a room which has a one-way mirror so that the meeting can be monitored by a second therapist. It is often helpful for the therapist to have a second person to discuss things with and also to pick up things she may have missed. Within a family the relationships can be so complex that one person cannot grasp what is going on. You will usually be asked if you would like to meet the person or persons behind the screen. If you are not offered this opportunity you are at liberty to ask. Some people object very strongly to the idea that they are being observed from behind the mirror, if you feel uncomfortable about it you should discuss your worries with the therapist. Most people forget that the mirror is there and are not upset by it.

Individual therapy

Opinions are divided about how useful individual therapy is for young children suffering from eating disorders. Research has shown that children who are given family therapy instead of individual therapy do better than those who have therapy alone. However no research has shown individual therapy to be harmful, so when done in conjunction with family therapy my view is that things can only be better. Certainly for those where the family situation is unlikely to change despite family work, individual therapy must have a major part to play. Again, there are endless discussions about whether or not very malnourished children can use individual therapy effectively. While I agree that there is no point in giving individual therapy to a child who is not being re-fed, I can see no harm in beginning the therapy as soon as re-feeding begins.

Group therapy

Some in-patient units run therapy groups for their children. It is sometimes easier for children to talk in a group than it is alone with a therapist. Others will find it hard to speak in a group but still derive some benefit from hearing what the others say.

In general, it would be true to say that anorexic patients are not ideally suited to working in groups and find it very difficult to interact. They are so worried about what people think of them, so sensitive to anything bordering on criticism that they find groups difficult to cope with and tend not to find them useful.

Marital therapy

Most family therapists are aware of the pressures an anorexic child puts on a marriage. Even if the marriage was rock solid before the child became ill, it is unlikely to be afterwards. All too often a child manages to split her parents; one is often wavering and finds it difficult to be firm while the other tries to take control. Anorexic children are expert at dividing people. Couples often row about the best approach to take, not realizing the opportunity this gives the child to get away with even more. The child aligns herself with one parent and a triangle is created.

The feelings of guilt and anxiety that an anorexic child brings are often too much for the strongest of marriages and conflict is common. Whilst the family therapist may be well aware of marital difficulties, she will probably only acknowledge them fleetingly and concentrate on the task in hand, i.e. of getting the child better.

As has already been mentioned, some children feel that their parents are only staying together because they are ill and that if they get better, their parents may separate. Parents have either to arrange to see the family therapist alone or to find a marriage counsellor who can support them. The child needs to know that her parents will make a decision to live together or separate, and that that decision will have nothing to do with their child's illness. In other words, whether the child is ill or well their decision will not be altered. Only when the parents can be clear about this will the child allow herself to get better.

Whether you are parents whose marriage is stable, a little shaky or you are already separated, you will have to find a way to work together to look after your child. Working together means agreeing about how she should be cared for and being consistent. Try not to let her split you and play one off against the other. Discuss your differences in private and present a united front.

Clinical psychologists

Parents are often confused about the difference between psychiatrists, psychologists and therapists. A psychiatrist is a medical doctor. She has done a five- or six-year general training and then worked for at least a year in a hospital as a general doctor. After that she has undertaken a training of at least seven years to become a psychiatrist, specialising in child psychiatry or adult psychiatry. The psychologist may be called a doctor but is not in fact a medical doctor. Psychologists have done a three-year degree course in psychology and then often carried on to study for a Ph.D. in clinical psychology which gives them a doctorate and the title of doctor. They are thus qualified to work with patients who have mental health problems.

Children who have severe obsessive-compulsive disorders or phobias are often seen by clinical psychologists. They sometimes see people with eating disorders.

Clinical psychologists are expert in helping people modify problem behaviours and in devising coping mechanisms for troubled children. They often use a form of therapy called cognitive behavioural therapy. This therapy involves the patient working with the therapist to question her beliefs and anxieties and examine her dysfunctional thoughts. They often have to monitor their eating and record her thoughts between sessions as an aid to discovering which sort of situation triggers an episode of binge eating. She might be asked to consider what evidence there is for her belief that she is fat or will become fat if she eats. This sort of therapy is particularly useful in treating people suffering from bulimia and is less frequently used for patients suffering from anorexia nervosa.

LINDA'S STORY

When Linda was eight years old her brother, our 10-year-old son, was knocked over and killed by a car as he was leaving school. We tried to hide our grief for Linda's sake. We were of course incredibly upset and never really got over his death. We kept his room exactly as it was, his toys and clothes still in his room as he had left it. Every year we went to France to the place where we had spent out last holiday together just before he died. We felt it was a sort of pilgrimage. We were very protective of Linda, we rarely let her out of our sight and she wasn't allowed to cross any roads or go on school trips. We explained to her that we loved her and didn't want her to have any accidents. I used to cry a lot and even four years after the accident I couldn't cope with thinking about him. When Linda was 12 she developed an eating disorder and needed to go into hospital which was traumatic for both of us. She had never been away from home before, even for a single night, and I didn't know how I was going to manage.

The family therapist we saw thought I was depressed and arranged for me to see someone myself. She started me on some antidepressants and after a couple of weeks I began to feel a bit better. I hadn't ever considered the effect David's death had had on Linda. We had all been trying to carry on as though nothing had happened when really we should have mourned him properly and then got on with our lives and looking after Linda. Soon after Linda came out of hospital we moved and I got a part-time job. It took Linda's illness to make us see that we all needed help. She just drew attention to it all.

Understanding the illness

If you are to help your child overcome her illness, you will have to be one jump ahead of her. You must know at least some of the tricks and have some understanding of her illness. Here is some vital background knowledge for your understanding of eating disorders. Don't be tempted to turn a blind eye and collude with her, it might make for a quiet life in the short term but in the long term it leaves her with no one to help her. She might be pushing to be in control, to decide about all aspects of her exercise and eating but deep down she is hoping that someone will make sensible decisions for her because she is too ill to make them herself. She will feel alone and helpless if her parents support her illness instead of the small part of her that wants to get better.

PERSONALITY CHANGES

Many anorexic children harbour a great deal of anger. What the anger is about can only be answered through therapy. This takes time and meanwhile the anger is often directed at her nearest and dearest. Sometimes their coldness towards their family is unexplained and sometimes there is a reason, such as making your child eat, insisting on her being weighed or admitting her to a unit against her will. While your child is refusing cuddles and acting in a hostile way it is difficult to continue being firm and tempting to give in to her so as not to inflame the situation. Tempting it might be, but wise it is not – anorexia must be treated by unyielding firmness and consistency. There is no room for giving in because 'my child might not love me anymore'. We all hear of children who have suffered terrible abuse at the hands of their parents and yet it is very clear that they still love their parents. The love that a child has for its parents is not a fragile love that can be easily destroyed. Insisting that your child does what you consider to be in her best interests and for the good of her health may evoke short-term annoyance but will not undermine their love for you. It is this idea, that a child's love can be lost forever if a parent makes a decision their child doesn't like, that leads so many parents to collude with their child's illness instead of helping her confront it.

Allowing your child to make the decision may buy you popularity today, but it could turn to resentment later, when she is left with the irreversible effects of having starved as a teenager.

Obsessive-compulsive disorders

Children with eating disorders are four times more likely to develop an obsessive-compulsive disorder than other children. We are not sure why this is the case. It may simply be due to the fact that these children are depressed and we know that obsessive-compulsive problems are exacerbated by depression.

Parents will often tell us that even before her illness, their daughter was a perfectionist. She liked everything to be very tidy, for example, the rows of bottles in the bathroom were arranged in order of height and the labels faced the same way. This perfectionist behaviour is not miles away from the more blatant obsessive-compulsive behaviour, which we see in many of our patients. They become anxious about cleanliness and germs, they wash their hands endlessly and change their clothes two or three times a day if unchecked. Many often become worried about walking on the cracks in the pavement and negotiate their way delicately along the road when out walking. Some of them develop rituals which they must perform, as they believe that something terrible will happen to them if they don't keep up the ritual. Some of these behaviours involve touching things or turning round before walking through a doorway. Many of the rituals we see are associated with eating, they pick, mash or spread their food, eat a sandwich in a certain pattern or pick the fillings out of pies.

These behaviours may be seen as harmless and not worthy of mention but they can actually cripple someone's life if they are allowed to go on unchecked. The best way to stop a ritual or compulsive behaviour is to encourage a child to stop and then realize that nothing terrible does in fact happen. All the time she is allowed to carry on performing these strange behaviours, she will feel the urge to do them more and more. If she can be stopped, the urge will gradually die off and she will at last find some peace of mind. You will have to be strong for her because she will have been taken over by the rituals. Initially she will feel extremely anxious about not being able to carry them out but try to distract her by other normal activities and her need to do them will fade. As she begins to eat normally and regain weight, her mood will lift and her obsessive-compulsive problems will be very much less prominent.

Body image

Body image is the mental image someone has of the way they look and the shape of their body. People suffering from anorexia nervosa and bulimia nervosa almost always have a distorted idea of their body shape. Sufferers are usually vomiting or restricting their food intake in the belief that they will improve their physical appearance. Body image dissatisfaction is extremely common amongst children and children as young as eight years old talk of their need to diet. A change in attitude to body image is vital if somebody is to recover from an eating disorder. A child with an eating disorder will frequently exaggerate her size and see herself as fat. Some children who have lost a lot of weight will realize that they are not fat and will be reasonably happy with their weight but will be sure that they will become ugly and unattractive if they gain weight.

Whether a distorted body image is a genuine phenomenon or a cover for their abnormal behaviour is difficult to tell. I have questioned many children who have recovered and they all say that they can remember very little about how they felt, or indeed if they felt. It seems that anorexia serves a useful purpose in deadening the mind and leaving little space for feelings. One thing I am sure of is that, when it comes to discussions about whether or nor anorexic children are fat or thin, the rational person cannot win. Frustrating as it may seem, one has to realize that one can argue, discuss, reason, or even demonstrate why an anorexic child is not fat and she will continue to hold steadfastly to the belief that she is fat. Parents very frequently ask us what they should do or say when their child appears to talk non-stop about how fat she is. Our advice is that one should not become embroiled in long and circuitous discussions about the relative size or fatness of arms, legs or tummies. It is a fruitless exercise which ends up making everyone cross. When you have a child of 13, for example, wearing children's clothes with age 9 on the label or a 15-year-old wearing size 10 trousers, it is obvious to any normal person that that child cannot be fat. The fact that you need to have the conversations is an indication that the child is not normal and most certainly needs professional help.

Depression

Most of the children admitted to our unit are suffering from depression and we know that a low-fat diet can cause depression. In most cases the depression leaves them once they are eating a normal and varied diet. Certainly very few children remain depressed once they have reached their target weight.

It is a common phase for anorexic children to go through and one can only reassure parents that this is a temporary phenomenon, which usually reverses as the child gets better. It is very common to hear that children who had previously been outgoing and sociable became withdrawn and quiet when they stopped eating. It is not always clear which came first, but eating properly and reaching a normal weight together with some psychiatric help is the only way in which the situation will improve. Most of the children we see remain popular. Their friends stick by them but during the acute phase of their illness they don't want to see their friends. They often spend long periods alone in their room studying. They often convince themselves that they are dull and boring and poor company. Be reassured that this is not a permanent problem; when your child recovers she will be the child you used to know.

Self-harm

Self-harm is relatively common among children who have eating disorders. Of all the injuries they inflict, cutting is probably the most usual. They sometimes cut their arms or legs where the cuts can be seen or in other cases they cut their breasts under their bra or their thighs where their injuries will not be noticed. Sometimes the injuries are very superficial and consist of a mass of scratches made with fingernails or sharp objects. They often pick at them so they do not heal. In some cases the cuts are deep and need extensive stitching. It is not unusual for self-harmers to remove their own stitches once they are home. In some cases children have burned themselves with lighters or on hot ovens. If you see burns, remember that sometimes the children are so cold that they accidentally burn themselves on radiators or hot water bottles in their attempts to keep warm. Other distressed children punch walls or hit their heads causing grazing and bruising. They often have very elaborate and almost plausible explanations for marks and injuries they have incurred. Be vigilant and check your child regularly if you have reason to be suspicious.

Children who cut or injure themselves explain that a tension builds up inside them with which they cannot cope. Cutting brings a release of that tension which temporarily relieves the stress they feel.

The ultimate form of self-harm is suicide or attempted suicide. Children with eating disorders, especially bulimic children, sometimes overdose on tablets. Most of the cases we have seen have taken reasonably small numbers of tablets and the children have told someone either immediately after or some time after ingesting them.

It does seem that, in the majority of cases, the children didn't really want to die, they wanted attention or they wanted to let people know how terrible they felt. The problem with these suicidal gestures is that children sometimes get it wrong. They either leave it too long before they tell someone or they take just a few too many tablets thinking that it wasn't very many.

Paracetamol is a particularly dangerous drug to take; some people are extremely sensitive to it. There have been cases of people taking only 12-15 tablets as a suicidal gesture and suffering liver damage, which has killed them.

If the child tells someone within two to three hours of taking the tablets she can be taken to hospital and have her stomach washed out. After this time much of the drug will have been absorbed. Aspirin in particular is absorbed very quickly from the stomach and a wash out needs to be done promptly.

It is not always overtly depressed children who harm themselves, they are very often not depressed at all but feeling completely hopeless. They are children who feel totally negative about their options, assuming that everything will turn out badly and unable to be anything other than pessimistic. They may have experienced one or more stressful life events or just feel that their life is in turmoil. Bulimic children especially tend to be impetuous and are most at risk of self-harming. If you suspect your child is self-harming, you should remove sharp knives from the kitchen, and razors and blades from the bathroom cupboard. Although these measures will make it harder for them to cut themselves, they will doubtless find other ways if they are determined. They use compass points, scissors or unscrew the blades from pencil sharpeners.

The only way to be sure that a child who is in this frame of mind doesn't cut is to be with her for 24 hours a day. At Rhodes Farm we search children's nightwear, bedding and books for hidden blades but from time to time can still miss the ones they have hidden in soft toys or in torches.

Talk to your daughter about the scarring that will never go and which will embarrass her for years to come when she wants to sit on a beach in a swimming costume. Most of the children who cut are too low in mood to be thinking about times when they might want to wear a sleeveless evening dress or sit on the beach. They can see no future, so your talk of scars will probably fall on deaf ears. Nevertheless, it is worth pointing out as she might think of it later, if not now. If you have a child with an eating disorder, do be careful not to leave tablets of any sort where she can find them. If she is taking antidepressant medication, make sure that she only has a few days' supply at a time. Tell your child about the dangers of paracetamol and how easy it is to misjudge the number of tablets in a cry-for-help type suicide attempt.

I will never forget when I was a junior doctor admitting a 16-year-old girl who had taken a paracetamol overdose. Two hours later she was sitting up in bed smiling and happy with her boyfriend sitting on her bed. She explained that they had had a row and that was why she had taken the tablets. She told me that everything was now fine. Later that evening her blood test showed that she had severe liver damage, which could not be treated. Three days later she died, a tragic waste of life, a suicidal gesture that went wrong.

Children who self-harm require urgent help. They need immediate referral to a therapist who can help them work through their problems. If it is thought that a child still feels as though she might harm herself, she should be referred for in-patient care so that she can be kept safe.

COMPULSIVE EXERCISING

Exercise often plays an integral part in the development of an eating disorder. There are several different types of compulsive exercising. In the first type the child openly exercises non-stop. She runs, swims and cycles several times a day and does the odd aerobics class or exercises in her room. She probably began with a gentle programme which she has had to increase bit by bit every day until she is taken over by her exercise. Many girls set their alarm clock for the middle of the night so that they can get up and exercise. They are never happy with what they achieve and always seek to improve their performance. I remember one parent telling me that her daughter used to cycle on her exercise bike for hours and she had even wet herself on several occasions rather than allow herself to stop. Some children who have always had a keen interest in a sport realize that in order to win and gain recognition they need to train more than anyone else. In the short term this inevitably brings the success they seek but some then decide to restrict their diet and avoid fat in the belief it will further enhance their performance. There is another group of anorexic children for whom exercise is undertaken purely for the effect it will have on speeding weight loss and not for any competitive motives. For whatever reason they begin to exercise the end result is much the same, an emaciated very weak child who by superhuman effort manages to push her frail body to the limit of human endurance.

CLARE'S STORY

Clare was a gifted sportswoman. She was 15 and was head of the netball team, captain of the tennis and hockey teams in the school swimming team and a long distance runner.

Despite the fact that she was very thin and was not having periods, she was never stopped from exercising because her parents thought 'it was too important to her'.

When she was admitted to our clinic we battled for four months to restore her weight and to bring her exercise under control. When we discharged her she was fit and well, exercising normally and just needing an adult to remind her every so often that she needed to take it easy.

Within three weeks of discharge, her parents had enrolled her in the local athletics club because the school was not allowing her to train properly. Her school had quite rightly taken advice from us and was helping her to keep her exercise to reasonable levels.

Six months later she was re-admitted to our clinic in an

extremely emaciated state and once again obsessed with exercising and standing up all day. She thought that she burnt off more calories standing than sitting and even did her school work standing up unless forced to sit down. Despite us explaining that she burnt off almost the same number of calories standing as sitting, she was more reluctant than ever to sit down and relax.

During her second stay we once again managed to curb her exercise and restore her weight and she was discharged home four months later.

Once again within two months of being at home she was training in the athletics club and playing in all the school teams. Her parents had threatened to move her from her private school if it tried to exclude her from games. Within six months she was admitted to another unit and spent the rest of her teenage years suffering from both anorexia and bulimia.

We once had two close friends from the same school resident in the clinic. They were inseparable and on the surface supported one another as best friends should. One evening, five minutes before the aerobics class began, one of the girls received a phone call telling her that her grandfather had died very unexpectedly. Her best friend put a hand on the shoulder of her sobbing friend and said 'I'll talk to you when I get back from aerobics' before shooting off so as not to miss a minute of her exercise. For children who exercise compulsively, relationships invariably take second place to exercise. We can think of many parents who having travelled 200 to 300 miles to visit their child, have been asked to accompany her to a swimming pool where they are expected to sit on the edge watching their single-minded son or daughter swim mindlessly up and down the pool. Exercise ceases to be a social activity which one does for fun and becomes a chore which has to be done, an obsession.

In the second type of compulsive exercising, the child still exercises endlessly but not so openly. She finds excuses to exercise and thinks that no one will notice. She will find different reasons to run upstairs and will constantly stand up instead of sitting down. She walks the dog five times a day and is extremely helpful in the home. She cleans, tidies, empties the dishwasher, cleans out the cupboards and sets the table. She is constantly on the go. Children like this who are never still manage to burn off a fair number of calories. Some children deprive themselves of sleep in the belief that they burn off more calories by being awake. It might be helpful to tell your child that she burns roughly 1 calorie a minute sleeping and 1.1 calories a minute awake in bed, not really a difference worth staying awake for. Similarly, she would use up about 1.5 calories a minute sitting and 2.1 calories a minute standing – the difference is negligible. However, when she is running up and down the stairs she burns off 6.5 calories a minute, which over a day can amount to several hundred calories being used up.

Many of the children who come to us are past the phase of being able to do lots of press-ups and exercise but nevertheless find it difficult to relax. This restlessness is difficult to overcome. It consists of constantly tapping the feet, flexing the leg muscles or moving the arms and it may be that they are not even aware that they are doing it.

Like all obsessions, the need for exercise becomes stronger the more the urge is given in to. Recovered anorexics will talk freely about how they were driven to exercise even when they were weak and dizzy. They begin by setting themselves a reasonable regime but gradually push themselves to do more and more. The urge is never satisfied. It compels them to do just a little more than last time. These children are no longer in charge of their actions, they are compulsively driven and need someone to stop them. Exercise puts added strain on a heart which is weakened by starvation, and they also risk damaging their joints through vigorous exercise as their damaged muscles are no longer able to support them adequately.

Over-exercising is one of the commonest reasons for a child who is apparently eating not to gain weight. You may notice your child rushing off to exercise immediately after a meal, in the mistaken idea that if she exercise quickly she can burn off the food she has just eaten before it can be laid down as fat. A little detective work is all that is needed to catch her, as the exercising is usually noisy. When prevented from exercising, as they must be if they are to recover, they may resort to climbing out of windows in the middle of the night and running for hours. The compulsive exerciser presents the same problem as a child who vomits, they need constant supervision night and day. Even in the bathroom they are likely to use the toilet as an aid to step-aerobics. Parents should not leave their children alone with this debilitating problem. It is not in their control, they cannot stop and they need you to put the brakes on.

Be firm

Parents are often prepared to make only a half-hearted effort to stop their children exercising. Of course it is difficult to stop a teenager and perhaps even more difficult to understand that something we would normally encourage can be so potentially damaging to a child with an eating disorder. The answer to children who just get on their bikes and cycle off is a very large padlock, and the way to stop other illicit exercise is large sanctions when caught or if rules are disobeyed.

If your child is a ballet dancer, swimmer or an athlete and cannot or will not eat enough food to keep up with the demands made by these activities, they must be stopped, not cut down but stopped altogether. No one under a safe weight should be doing more than a little gentle exercise. Cycling, dancing, running and racing in a swimming pool should be stopped until a safe weight has been reached. They can then be resumed gradually but stopped again immediately the child slips even ½kg below target weight. Compulsive exercising is usually aimed at speeding weight loss. It becomes much less of a problem once a child reaches a target weight and understands that she must stay there.

There must be no negotiation, no second chances – you must stick rigidly to your rules if you are to succeed. A child who is given a second chance will feel duty-bound to push a little further to see if there will be a third or even a fourth chance. Remember that children thrive on having boundaries and rules that they can rely on. You may think you are being kind but in fact the child becomes confused and unsure about how to interpret what you say. A child is more likely to be upset and angry if you suddenly impose rules having given her three or four chances than if you act immediately the rule is breached.

Children do not need to work out, jog or swim endlessly in order to keep fit. It is recommended that normal healthy children and adults exercise for about 20 minutes three times a week. Of course most children do more than this as part of their school curriculum. Only athletes need to do more than this and their training should be supervised and sensibly worked out by a qualified coach. Many of the children we see are doing more exercise than Olympic athletes in training. Of course, the more exercise you do, the more you have to eat; some athletes eat between 5,000 and 6,000 kcal a day.

THE EFFECTS OF ANOREXIA NERVOSA

It is a good idea to make sure that your child is aware of the terrible consequences of poor eating. It may be that like so many children I see, your child takes little notice. She will think either it will never happen to her or that it does not apply to her because she doesn't see that she is ill. However, I have seen children whose attitudes have completely changed when they have been made aware of how they are damaging their bodies. To understand the long- and short-term effects of anorexia nervosa will also help you realize how important it is to help your child battle against her illness and not give up. It is not enough to simply raise her weight to a level where she is out of immediate danger. In some cases after only a few years at sub-normal weight some of the irreversible side-effects of starvation can be seen.

Short-term effects

The short-term effects of anorexia nervosa are usually apparent within a few weeks of starvation beginning. In girls, their periods stop very early on, sometimes before vast quantities of weight have been lost. When pre-pubertal girls starve, sexual development is arrested and there is no development of breasts, ovaries or uterus. In children who have reached puberty, periods stop and their ovaries and uterus shrink. Children who do not eat properly do not grow and if starvation occurs before puberty and the growth spurt then they remain stunted by their illness. Most children who are limiting their food intake are depressed, which is thought to be caused by a lack of fat. Similarly, a low fat diet causes poor concentration and interferes with memory.

Children with anorexia often develop a fine downy hair on their back and face. It is unsightly and children need to know that their poor eating habits have caused it.

As starvation continues muscles become affected by the malnutrition and major nerves no longer protected by a fat layer become prone to pressure damage. The result of this is severe muscle weakness which can prevent that patient walking properly.

It is very common for children who do not eat to faint or feel dizzy. This is due to the fact that their heart is not pumping as efficiently as it should and they have very low blood pressure. This is particularly noticeable when they stand up quickly.

Many children who do not eat properly develop anaemia. This is due to their poor diet often lacking meat and iron. Anaemia causes tiredness and in some cases affects the heart. It is reversed very quickly once the child begins to eat a normal diet and weight is restored.

Children who have starved for long periods of time often complain of feeling extremely full or bloated or of having pains in their tummy when they are asked to eat. Usually this is quite unrelated to any physical problems and is simply a psychological affect. Not surprisingly, prolonged starvation does affect the digestive system and sometimes when a child begins to eat again she does find that her stomach remains full for longer than normal or that she is constipated. These problems resolve as the body gradually becomes accustomed to normal amounts of food again.

Children have a smaller percentage of body fat than adults and thus become ill much sooner when they begin to lose weight. One early sign of impending problems is a low pulse rate and low blood pressure. Despite these easily recordable measures of ill health, we see many, many children who are at dangerously low weights, having seen a psychiatrist or psychologist once a week but not having had their pulse and blood pressure taken regularly. The outwards signs of starvation are clear to see: bones and veins which protrude through skin which has no underlying fat and muscle wasting. It is vital that your child is given regular physical examinations so that any problems can be identified early and treated quickly.

Long-term effects

If periods and normal development are arrested long term, there is considerable risk of infertility. In our experience it is relatively easy to restore a normal menstrual cycle in girls whose loss of periods is less than two years, providing they can be held at a good weight. The longer the time without periods the longer it takes to restore them. Unfortunately, we have several children who have been at target weight for three years and still have not menstruated. Loss of periods is a very worrying confirmation that dieting has got out of hand and should be taken very seriously. It is not acceptable to leave children who are not menstruating at low weights. In girls who develop the illness before puberty it is even more vital that they are restored to normal weight and reach puberty before any permanent damage is done.

Another serious problem caused by abnormal hormone levels is that of osteoporosis. In osteoporosis, the bones are not as dense as they should be and they fracture very easily, or, more seriously, the vertebrae can collapse causing damage to the spinal cord. In children eating a normal diet, their bones gain more calcium than they lose every day until their early twenties. They should have reached their maximum density by this time because, from then on, calcium loss outstrips gain even before menopause, when the loss is then greatly speeded up. Taking calcium supplements has no effect on the rate of bone loss as the calcium cannot be absorbed without eostrogen. Even when there is oestrogen being produced, its effectiveness is dependent on there being a certain percentage of body fat, for it is within the fat that oestrogen is metabolised. Athletes who may have a body weight which is in theory sufficient for normal menstruation, commonly do not have periods and develop osteoporosis due to their low body fat. Even though it is rare for teenagers to develop fractures, any bone loss at this stage will inevitably increase the risk of bone problems later on.

As well as the wrist and hip fractures which commonly occur in osteoporotic patients after even a relatively minor accident, the vertebrae often collapse causing an ugly dowager's hump which we have all seen.

The important fact that should be understood by girls and boys who diet excessively is that the damage done to the bone is not always reversible as the calcium deficit is not always made up, even when they begin to eat normally again. There have been reports of children developing osteoporotic fractures as little as one year after stopping their periods. Boys are also at risk of osteoporosis when they diet as their testosterone levels drop in much the same way as oestrogen in girls.

When the body becomes very cold through lack of food, the small blood vessels in the hands and feet constrict so that less blood flows through the fingers and toes and heat is conserved. This shutting down restricts the circulation and the extremeties become blue and icy cold. If this situation continues, the tissues in the toes and fingers receive so little blood, and therefore oxygen, that they begin to die. Dead tissue very quickly becomes blocked and gangrenous and there have been several reported cases of children whose feet have been affected in this way. There are many long-term anorexic patients who have needed below knee amputations because of the damage to their blood vessels.

The psychological problems

We are not sure whether a low self-esteem is something which causes an eating disorder or whether it is caused by an eating problem but, whichever way round it is, it is a very common problem with teenagers with eating disorders. Self-esteem is a difficult notion to explain. It is to do with the way we value ourselves as people and the way we regard ourselves. Anorexic children often do not feel good about themselves, they feel that nothing they do is good enough and they are easily upset. Other children may weather the same knocks that life doles out such as parents divorcing, bereavement, even abuse, without it affecting their self-esteem. Anorexic children tend to be more delicate; they have a far less robust attitude to life.

This lack of self-esteem can take many forms. They may think that they are hopeless students and that the world will come to an end if they don't achieve grade As. Their perfectionist traits also play a part here. Many anorexic children work excessively on their schoolwork but they need to understand that starvation affects their ability to concentrate and to study effectively. They would be wiser and would certainly work more efficiently if they ate normally and put in fewer hours. One cannot expect a starved brain to retain facts and do its best. The brain is dependent upon a constant supply of glucose in order to function properly. Although it cannot be denied that starving children usually achieve excellent grades in examinations, it does involve superhuman efforts which probably would not be necessary if they were not starving.

Anorexic children often think that no one likes them. In their pursuit of perfection they want 'perfect' friends and become unhappy if this is not the case. This often means that they devote a lot of time to one particular person and inevitably sooner or later feel let down. It is extremely difficult to live up to the high standards that these children set for themselves, their friends and their family.

Sometimes they feel that no one likes them because their friends have given up calling them. Their friends do stop calling simply because they realize that the child never wants to join in with their activities. Anorexic children who do not like themselves often feel that they lack personality or intelligence or make boring company. They envy their friends who are more outgoing and feel that being ultra-thin will in some way compensate for their lack of social graces. Many of these children have been the victim of bullying and this adds fuel to the idea that they are worthless individuals.

Lack of growth

Another feature of starvation, which is important in children, is lack of growth. We commonly see children who have been stunted by years of malnutrition and who are unlikely ever to reach their full growth potential. Children who do not grow or develop normally do not look abnormal during their teens as people just presume they are younger than their years. However, this situation changes as they enter their twenties. Very short people whose normal development has been arrested take on a bizarre elfin look, boys' voices do not break, and these unhappy people usually lead a lonely life.

In most cases, children who have fallen behind with their growth grow very rapidly once they begin to eat a good diet. It is not unusual for us to see children grow 2–3 cm in a few weeks while in the clinic. However, this stops again immediately if they fall below their target weight. It must be remembered that although the children do start to grow again, they may not catch up fully.

Similarly, breast development will probably never reach its full potential once stopped by a period of starvation.

THE MEDICAL CONSEQUENCES OF VOMITING

Your child needs to know about the risks she takes when she vomits. Many people find it hard to believe that teenagers and adults alike can die very suddenly from the effects of vomiting.

The rhythmic beating of our heart is dependent on there being a constant and finely controlled balance of sodium and potassium in our body. The intestine and stomach act as a reservoir for potassium and when people vomit or abuse laxatives they lose large quantities of potassium, which then disrupts the heartbeat. When the potassium falls too low these people can have heart attacks and die, even though their weight is not low and they neither look nor feel particularly ill. It is for this reason that we say that children who persistently vomit should be admitted to hospital, as it is not safe for them to be at home. They need to have their blood potassium levels monitored and to be prevented from vomiting. Children will always listen politely to the grave complications of vomiting and often think that it will never happen to them – they need to be persuaded that it could.

CHAPTER FIVE

What to expect from a specialist unit

If you have not been able to help your child gain weight at home, do not despair. Trying to treat your own child is never easy and often children need to be away from home. Many of the mothers who bring their children to us are very aware of the abnormally enmeshed and clingy relationship which has developed since their child became ill and they recognize the need for some independence and separation.

You have not failed because your child needs to be admitted to hospital. Some children need the more specialised care they receive there. It will give you a chance to recharge your batteries. Although your child should be physically well and much better by the time she is discharged, it is unlikely that she will be fully cured and will certainly be in need of your help again.

PARENTS IN CONTROL

If your child is damaging her body, her long-term health and her education through self-starvation, this is clearly a situation which cannot be allowed to continue. It is obvious that anyone who is very thin and ill, and is refusing to eat, is not thinking normally and is not in a position to make rational decisions. For this reason, she needs responsible people to be in charge of her and to make the right decisions for her. I often feel that some of the patients we see have reached the stage they are at because they don't have people who are strong enough to make these decisions on their behalf. I feel that too much responsibility is often placed on the sick child. She is asked all too often for her consent and co-operation, consent which she cannot give because her illness has taken her over and is much stronger than she is. There is always the little part of every anorexic child that wants to get better, but that part is easily stifled by the illness which overpowers her with guilt should she even think about eating and putting on weight.

People often ask me how it is that we get the children in our clinic to eat. We do it through being firm and taking responsibility away from the child. She has to eat, there is no way around it and under these circumstances she can relax, pick up a knife and fork and eat without feeling guilty.

Leaving a child alone with her illness by allowing her to choose whether to eat, whether to exercise or whether to vomit is cruel. She might be pushing you to allow her to choose but deep down she is hoping that someone will just tell her what to do.

Most anorexic children are seeking to take control but when they realize that in fact they are in charge of everything, their life, their parents, they panic and feel very insecure. Children much prefer to have parents who are in charge.

I often see parents and professionals who think that when a child is 16 she can no longer be forced to accept treatment. Thankfully, this is not the case. She cannot refuse treatment and she cannot discharge herself from a hospital. The law states that, 'No minor of whatever age (a minor being under 18 years old) has the power by refusing to consent to treatment, to override a consent to treatment by any one who has parental responsibility for the minor.'

In a case in 1992 the appeal court ruled that a 19-year-old girl with anorexia nervosa had no absolute right to refuse medical treatment in circumstances when refusal to accept such treatment might cause severe harm. In this case the court was told that irreversible damage to her brain and reproductive organs would ensue if she refused food.

It is clearly not the case that we have to sit by and watch a child's weight continue to drop because we don't have the permission to treat her.

Even if your child is over 18, you can try and make decisions for her which are in her best interests. An 18-year-old usually still needs her parents to provide her with a roof over her head and a grant or pocket money. In these circumstances she is not in a position to call the shots and decide whether or not to discharge herself from hospital. You are in a very strong position and simply have to point out that if she is to discharge herself you will not be responsible for her. If indeed she is claiming to be an independent adult who makes her own decisions, she needs it pointed out to her that she can also find herself somewhere to live and some way of supporting herself. If your daughter sees that you mean what you are saying, she is likely to stay where she is. Do not be tempted to waiver.

We occasionally have cases referred to us where despite the fact that the child is very ill, her parents do not feel that the situation is serious enough to warrant an admission to hospital. In these cases, social services usually make an application for the child to be made a ward of court, and the guardian can then give permission for treatment.

Your child's rights

Children are especially at risk if they develop an eating disorder as their bodies store less fat than adults. They therefore become ill very quickly and often need urgent treatment. The majority of children we treat do not want to be treated and some even say they want to die.

Depriving the brain of nutrients stops it functioning normally and this needs to be taken into account when deciding whether or not these children are competent to make decisions. We see very starved children who take half an hour to decide which chocolate bar to take or which chair to sit on, so to make life and death decisions about treatment would certainly be too much for them.

In 1989 the Children's Act was passed. It is a law which tries to allow children some say in decisions which effect them. The Act states that the wishes of the child should be taken into consideration when reaching a decision but in the light of their age and ability to understand. It is not an Act that gives children the right to do what they like, although it is sometimes misinterpreted in this way.

Children should be consulted and asked for their views on a subject such as hospital treatment but the ultimate decision must take into account whether the child's wishes are compatible with what is thought by adults to be in her best interests. In one of his High Court hearings Lord Donaldson made a very clear statement about anorexia nervosa. He said '...it is a feature of anorexia nervosa that it is capable of destroying the ability to make an informed choice. It creates a compulsion to refuse treatment or only to accept treatment which is likely to be ineffective. This attitude is part and parcel of the disease and the more advanced the illness the more compelling it may become.'

In cases involving minors suffering from anorexia nervosa the compulsory treatment would usually involve not only obliging the child to stay in the unit but to agree to eat or be fed by a naso-gastric tube if necessary.

Despite the fact that the Children's Act provides us with the legislation to treat children against their will if necessary, there are still many professionals who advocate treating children as adults and using the Mental Health Act as a way forward if they refuse treatment which is deemed necessary. For people detained under the Mental Health Act there are many. It is often something asked about on job application forms and insurance policy forms. Under the Mental Health Act two doctors and a mental health care professional decide whether or not a person is suffering from a mental illness and requires compulsory treatment. Treating children under this Act is like using a sledge-hammer to crack a nut. It is neither necessary nor advisable.

Don't waste time

Children who are underweight do not grow, and their lack of periods (with low hormone levels) causes permanent damage to their bones and they risk infertility. Those of us who work with these children all agree that we cannot allow them to damage themselves in this way. Sick children cannot be expected to make decisions about whether or not they want to be treated. It falls to parents to make difficult decisions such as this on behalf of their child. It is surprising how long some parents wait before agreeing to admit their children for treatment of this life-threatening disease.

When you have exhausted every avenue open to you as an out-patient and done everything you can to keep your child at home, you are left with little choice but to seek help from professionals, skilled and experienced at helping anorexic children to eat. You cannot shirk the responsibility of making this decision even though it is very unlikely to meet with the approval of your child. Your child could well die before she sees the necessity of asking for help. If you are not able to make your child eat enough food to gain a minimum 1kg a week, you are failing her by keeping her at home.

We have met many parents who have wasted months and in some cases years of their child's young life, always giving her one last chance and believing her promises to eat tomorrow. It is reasonable to have one attempt at a plan such as the one suggested in this book but if it fails, admit defeat and seek help sooner rather than later. The prognosis for recovery is much better for children with a short history.

Any child whose weight-for-height ratio is below 80 per cent needs to be in hospital if she is not gaining weight consistently at home. Once a child's periods stop she begins losing calcium from her bones every day. This calcium loss will never be recovered and the bones will never reach their maximum density. We have seen teenagers whose periods have stopped for only a year, with poorly calcified bones which fracture easily.

However ill and weak she becomes, your child will tell you that she feels fit and well. She will probably demonstrate this fact by running everywhere and continuing to take part in several sports, but do not take this as evidence of her good health. Anorexic children exercise to the point of collapse; they will never admit that they are struggling.

A cry for help

Inside your child will be feeling anxious and alarmed by the fact that her illness is out of control. She will be silently crying out for help and hoping someone will relieve her of the responsibility of coping alone with this terrifying illness.

As well as food poorly hidden in her room, she may leave you other clues such as diaries left open and prominently displayed. It is fair to say that a diary left open on a bed or table has been left there deliberately in the hope that someone will read it. What you read will need some interpretation. It may be a cry for help or a veiled threat such as her plan to commit suicide if you thwart her wishes. Suicide threats are very common amongst this group of very sick children, as are threats to run away. Many parents refrain from doing what they know to be in their child's best interests for fear of her carrying out her threat to run away or kill herself. Our advice to parents who face this dilemma is not to give in to emotional blackmail of this type. Once you have given in to threats such as these, your child will have total control and you will have none. She will be able to use the same tactics to persuade you to reverse any future decisions you may make.

Very few children are in a position to run away. They rarely have anywhere to go and receive no help from social services until they are 18. Despite repeatedly hearing these threats from the children in our care, we have never had a single case of a child joining the down-and-outs under Waterloo Bridge, which seems to be their parents' greatest fear.

As for committing suicide, it is unlikely that your child is suicidal, but if she was it would probably provide you with an even stronger reason for making the decision she opposes so much. Children who make attempts on their life very rarely do it following threats of this sort. Of course there are no guarantees that your child will not carry out her threat, but what is sure is that you cannot let this behaviour prevent you doing what you know to be right. If you stand by your decision regardless of threats, you may well have to weather a tantrum but it will probably be followed by a calm resignation that can only be described as relief. Relief that, at last, she no longer needs to fight her illness alone.

CHOOSING THE RIGHT IN-PATIENT TREATMENT FOR YOUR CHILD

If your clinician has recommended in-patient treatment, you now need to decide where that will be. Anorexic children can be treated in one of four different places. The first and perhaps the most common place to treat a child with anorexia nervosa is on a paediatric ward. If the child is acutely ill due to dehydration or malnutrition then the general doctors on the paediatric ward will be able to re-hydrate her and feed her for a few days in order to stabilise her physical symptoms. The paediatric ward is the ideal place for a child who needs urgent medical treatment but it is certainly not the right place for a child with a psychiatric illness and who needs long term refeeding. Usually, although of course there are exceptions, the general nurses on paediatric wards know very little about anorexia and are not experts in encouraging children to eat. Paediatric wards are for children with short-term illnesses, they are not designed for long stay patients. In many paediatric wards, the schooling is poorly organised and therapy and family meetings are not always available.

The Royal College of Psychiatrists published in 1992 a recommendation that children with eating disorders be treated in specialised units. Unfortunately there are not enough of these to go round. Some child and adolescent psychiatric units, whilst not dedicated solely to the treatment of children with eating disorders, do have some nurses who are experienced with these types of problems. These units also admit children who have behavioural problems or who are depressed, and if these children present more challenging behaviours than the anorexic or bulimic children, they are of necessity given more attention. Anorexic children are usually withdrawn, sad children who are often very academic, and their needs can be overlooked on a busy child and adolescent unit.

Specialist units

Where possible you should try to insist that your child is treated in a unit which specialises in helping children with eating disorders. The staff will have a vast experience of refeeding children, they will know all the tricks of the trade and more importantly will be more understanding of the illness and the way your child is feeling. Some people argue that it is not a good idea to put a lot of anorexic children together, saying that they learn to be better anorexics and that others will lead them astray. In my experience the opposite is true. It is very much easier to encourage children to eat and put on weight when exposed to the peer pressure of a group. In our clinic, there are very positive benefits to be gained from achieving a 1kg-a-week weight gain and the majority of the group are working towards doing that. They also derive a lot of help from being surrounded by other children who are struggling with the same illness. Anorexic children are usually very supportive and very caring. There are always children in the group who are getting better and are positive enough to be of real help to newcomers. In a good unit, the children are not trying to learn ways of avoiding putting on weight, they are working to keep on course and looking forward to reaching their various goals. In my opinion the advantages of treating children with eating disorders in specialised groups far outweigh any disadvantages.

Adult psychiatric units

The one place that you should never allow your child to go is to an adult psychiatric unit or an adult eating disorders unit. Even a 16- or 17-year-old is too young to be with women who are chronically ill. Many of the patients on adult psychiatric units have been ill for a very long time and are certainly poor company for someone with a relatively short history. Another drawback of adult units is that they often have a regime which allows for the fact that the majority of the patients will be looking after themselves and living independently when they leave. In treating teenagers the emphasis is on putting the parents back in charge, a completely different emphasis from that needed for adults.

Adult units do not usually provide full-time schooling, which is vital for most teenagers who do not want to add to their problems by getting behind at school.

One final reason for not admitting your child to an adult unit is that many of her fellow patients will smoke, some of them very heavily.

LIFE IN A SPECIALIST UNIT

Once in the unit, your child will be learning to eat normally again and steadily gaining weight. She will be panicked not only by having to put on weight but also by no longer being able to eat salads and low-fat foods. Your child will almost certainly want to leave soon after admission, even if it was her choice to be admitted. Having to eat previously 'forbidden' foods like chips and cheese comes as a shock and her immediate reaction will be to leave. She will probably telephone you and tell you how unhappy she is. Knowing that having to eat pizza and cream cakes is not going to evoke any sympathy from you, she will choose other ways of persuading you that this is not the right place for her to be. She is aware that she is more likely to tug at your heart strings by telling you that none of the staff and patients like her, that she has no one to talk to and that she cries herself to sleep every night. You must make up your own mind about the unit she is in. Discuss any worries about her being constantly upset or lonely with the staff. You will probably find that she is only upset when she talks to friends and relatives. It usually takes a week or two for a new patient to settle in and then the worrying phone calls and letters should start to tail off. Try to avoid the inevitable pleas about lowering her target weight. She is unlikely to accept the necessity of reaching this weight and any discussions about it are fruitless. Almost all our patients tell their parents that they have no intention of staying at their target weight on discharge and most of them are extremely angry with their parents for at least the first two weeks of admission. If the unit runs a parent support group, you will find it helpful to meet other parents who are experiencing or have experienced similar problems. If there is not a formal group, ask the staff to put you in contact with other parents who have been through the same thing.

SUE'S STORY

We had Sue admitted to an eating disorders unit when she was 13; she was very thin. She was very reluctant to go and made us promise that we would take her out before she got to her target weight as she thought it sounded too much. We did a deal with her and said that as long as she ate and was good, we would take her home when she had put on half the weight and she could put on the rest at home.

She hated the unit, she didn't make friends, she didn't like anyone and never settled in. She told the other girls that we had agreed to take her out after a few weeks and the nurses heard about it too. We had to admit to the staff that we had promised to take her out early but we were already beginning to regret our promise as she was doing well weight-wise and we didn't want to upset things. We didn't need a lot of persuading by the staff to change our minds and we very reluctantly told Sue that we were not going to do as we had promised. She was furious with us, she screamed and ranted and slammed doors but we held firm. The next morning she absconded from the unit and we had no idea where she had gone. We spent a very anxious day worrying about what could have happened to her. Eventually at about 6pm she rang us up from a station and we went to collect her. We decided to return her immediately to the unit and not home as she was begging us to do.

The staff explained to us that Sue had never attempted to settle in or make friends because not only was it a waste of time because she would soon be leaving, but she also needed us to see that she was unhappy and wanted to come home. Our promise to discharge her early gave her no motivation at all to settle in and take part in things. Once we told her that we had changed our minds and were breaking our promise to discharge her early, she became so angry that she ran away.

Once she got over the shock of knowing that she had to stay, she relaxed and began to join in with the other children. We are clear that we should have been firmer from the start.

The Rhodes Farm way

Depending on which establishment your daughter finds herself in, the regime will vary enormously. At Rhodes Farm, even if we knew or could understand what caused or triggered the development of anorexia nervosa in a particular child, it not not help at all in putting us in any better position to help the child recover. Very often, by the time a child comes for treatment, the reason or causes of her first developing the illness are long past. They may even have been resolved and forgotten. What is important when we first meet a family is to decide where we go from here. Looking backwards, especially apportioning blame, is a futile exercise. We are faced with a sad child who cannot eat with her family. Whatever triggered this illness can be very different from what is currently maintaining it and preventing her from getting better. We have to appreciate that the starvation itself now adds to her problems.

In the war, there were experiments carried out on volunteers which involved them being put on a very low-calorie semi-starvation diet. The effects were studied and monitored. The volenteers reported many disturbances, among them, loss of appetite, irritability, emotional instability, depression and lack of concentration. So, we can see that dieting alone could well be contributing to a lot of the psychological disturbances we see in these children. This, together with concerns for her physical health, is an overwhelming reason for ensuring quick and effective weight gain.

On paediatric wards and in some adolescent units, there may be very little emphasis put on food and eating. I'm never very sure why this is. It may because they don't understand the serious consequences of the child staying at a low weight. It may be that they do not have the expertise to feed the child and cover this by saying that food is not an issue. I happen to think that food is very important, it is in fact the main reason that a child is taken away from home and put into a unit. The child is not there just to have therapy, she can have individual and family therapy at home. She is in a unit because she doesn't eat and her physical condition has deteriorated to a dangerous level. As far as I am concerned if someone is going to recommend that your child leaves your family because you are unable to persuade her to eat, and her weight has become critical, they must be able to do better than you. The very least you should expect from a unit which is supposed to be caring for anorexic children is that your child gains weight steadily. If she does not, you must question the use of her being there.

Many good units will have a refeeding regime whereby your child will begin by eating smallish meals to get her accustomed to eating again. After a few days they will gradually increase her intake until she is able to gain 1kg per week steadily. This will probably mean altering the amount of calories she eats regularly. Her metabolism will increase and her activity level will also go up as she begins to feel better.

It is important that your child is given proper food and not liquid food supplements as she should be working towards normal eating. For teenagers, normal eating includes such things as chips, hamburgers, pizza and chocolate. She should be encouraged while she is in the unit to eat normal food and not to try to avoid fatty foods like cheese, chips and chocolate.

In an in-patient unit you should expect your child to be given a full day of schooling from Monday to Friday. Your child will probably be very concerned about her school work and will not want to fall behind.

Some units expect children to stay on their beds for several hours following a meal, this is to prevent them from vomiting or over-exercising. This is not something we do at Rhodes Farm; we supervise the children but would not ask them to remain inactive. We are extremely keen that the children in our care should be kept occupied and not left to worry about their weight gain or what horrors the next meal will bring. Exercise is the normal healthy part of the child's day and as long as it is not becoming a compulsive problem should be continued while the child is gaining weight. Doing a little walking or swimming or playing a game of rounders or badminton does not make a major difference to the amount of food that a child has to eat in order to gain weight. At Rhodes Farm the children are allowed to do a normal amount of exercise as long as they are gaining the required amount. If the weight gain drops off, then the child has to realize that all her exercise has to stop until the deficit has been made up. Equally, if we find that children are exercising in secret, the normal activities which we allow are stopped to compensate for the clandestine exercising.

Setting a target weight

A target weight is generally regarded as being the lowest weight at which a child can function, grow and develop normally. Research carried out at Great Ormond Street Hospital for Sick Children has shown that for the majority of girls this weight should be set at 5 per cent below the average weight for children of the same age and height. For boys who have a much lower percentage of body fat, we prefer to set the target weight at the average weight, not below it.

The results show that below this weight a child's body is very unlikely to function normally. Above it, hormone levels return to normal and in girls this is characterised by the return of her periods.

Re-establishing periods and growth have to be top priority in treating anorexic children. If the child's weight can be restored and held at a safe level, one buys time for the longer process of healing her mind. Although some children recover quickly once treated, others need months or sometimes years of ongoing psychiatric help. Being at a healthy weight gives a child the best possible chance of recovery. She will feel well, be growing and menstruating, keeping up at school and at home with her friends and family. We so often see children in their late teens who are so physically damaged by their illness and who have missed so much school that they have little chance of a normal life. Parents owe it to their anorexic child at least to see that she is not left with a legacy of ill health. We cannot heal their minds without their co-operation but we need no such consent to heal their bodies. Time is not on our side when a child's development is arrested; there is no place for non-interventionist methods.

A target weight is easily calculated using a standard rule incorporating data used by all paediatricians. As far as our clinic is concerned, the target weight is absolutely non-negotiable. We make no concession to mythical ideas about light bones, small bones or small frames, as children's growth charts take account of only age, height and weight. Only if periods return before target weight and the child has a normal amount of body fat do we reduce the target weight. If children do not reach a safe weight, not only do they risk ill health but there is evidence to suggest that it is more difficult to keep them at a sub-optimum weight when hormone levels are still abnormal than it is at a correct weight. It would be fair to say that, almost without exception, anorexic children do not accept the need to achieve a target weight, or at least not the target weight that we set. Most anorexics have their own 'target weight' based on being about a stone lighter than the thinnest person they know. Hearing the weight we expect them to attain fills them with panic and any good intentions they may have had about wanting to get better are temporarily abandoned. They often rant and rave and many announce their intention of losing all the weight again as soon as they are discharged home.

The shock is made worse by the fact that some of our patients have been set totally unrealistic target weights by their previous units. As far as we can tell, they were arrived at by a combination of what the patient would like to weigh and the size of her grandmother's bones. Certainly science has had little part to play in the calculation of most of these goal weights. Whilst we expect and understand that our anorexic patients would not need admission if they were eager and willing to munch their way to our target weight, we never cease to be amazed by how many parents also try to negotiate the weight we set. One parent discharged his child prematurely from the clinic because he had seen her in a swimming costume and in his opinion 'she had a lovely little figure'. Like his daughter, his only concern was for what she looked like, with no thought of her long-term health.

As professionals we need your support. Our job becomes impossible if we find ourselves in conflict with both child and parents. When this does happen, the illness invariably gets the upper hand. When the target weight is reached, we find a vast number of parents, who having co-operated all the way, no longer see the need to insist on the weight being maintained. The weight we set is a minimum weight. If it was safe to be 1kg below it, we would have set the target 1kg lower. It is very confusing for children who have been pressurised into reaching a specific weight, suddenly to find that it is no longer important whether they stay at it or a kilogram or two below it. Anorexic children respond very well to consistency and will usually accept the inevitable. This is yet another case of where one must set rules and stick to them. If you allow her to drop 1 or 2kg she will soon be pushing for 3 or 4kg lower and then 5 or 6kg. She will never be happy.

Target weights are not set for life. It is very important that you and your child understand that normal children gain weight continuously until the ages of 16 to 18 when they have completely stopped growing. Between the ages of 11 to 12 and 12 to 13 the average child gains about 5 kg. Children who have not grown because of a poor diet quite often catch up dramatically when they begin eating and their target weight needs to be revised every two to three months. If you do not measure your child regularly you can find that she has dropped to a dangerously low percentage again even though she has not actually lost weight.

Parents who are unhappy about the target weight we have set often tell us it is too high because 'she has never been that weight before'. We try to explain, although not always success-fully, that they are comparing her target weight with the weight she was a year or more ago and that, had she not developed anorexia nervosa, she would have gained 5 to 6kg during that time. It is therefore true to say that she has never been that weight before but nevertheless it is the weight she would have been if her illness had not intervened.

Children are very quick to realize the significance of having periods and the fact that if they menstruate before reaching their target weight it might be lowered. If your daughter claims to have started her periods below her target weight, you will have to verify this before allowing her to stablilise her weight. At our clinic we give the girls a new sanitary towel and do not let them out of our sight for two hours. We then check the pad. We used to content ourselves with a glance at the soiled towel but when we found out that the girls were collecting used pads from the toilets of the local squash club, we decided to be more vigilant. Parents are often very indignant about us not simply accepting their daughter's word, but experience has taught us not to take anything at face value.

If you feel unable to intrude on her privacy in the way that doctors and nurses can, you can verify that she is menstruating by asking your GP to refer her for an ultrasound scan of her uterus and ovaries. This is a very simple non-intrusive investi-gation, exactly the same as performed on pregnant women. It will quickly confirm that her ovaries and uterus are functioning normally and it is safer for her to stay at her current weight.

Communication

At Rhodes Farm, and probably at other units, the number of telephone calls you and your child may have will be limited. We do this because it is easier for the child to settle in when she can't constantly run to you with every tiny problem. If she has problems in the unit, it is much better that she discusses them with the other children or the staff instead of passing them on to you. If you are always on call, she will tell you about her problems instead of those in the unit who are better placed to help her with them. She must build relationships with her peers and her nurses and this is much easier for her to do if she is away from you. Another reason we limit telephone calls is that if we let the children initiate calls to their parents whenever they want, they will almost always choose to call when things are going badly. If she has just had to eat a big meal and is feeling fat and full, that is the time when she will phone you to pour out all her frustrations and anxieties. You are probably not the best person to help her with her feelings and, secondly, she will leave you feeling worried and helpless. We often have telephone calls from parents pleading with us to go and find their child who has just been crying on the phone to them and has left them with the impression that she is suicidal. We scurry off to find the child and usually discover her sitting in the lounge happily playing with the play station with her friends.

If your child writes you letters telling you she wants to die or is going to run away, do share this with the staff of the unit as it is very important that they know how your child is feeling. They may be totally unaware that there is a crisis looming. If your child should run away, try not to panic. We frequently have children absconding from our unit but in 10 years no one has ever come to any harm. Most children run home and a few just walk around for a bit then return to the unit. One thing you must do is resist any temptation to enter into deals with your child should she telephone you. Make it clear to her that she will be returned to the unit the second she walks in your door. She will not be allowed to stay overnight or to make herself at home, she will be taken back immediately. If you tell her this will happen and then do it, it is unlikely that she will run away again.

Not surprisingly, most children are very unhappy during their first week or two in a unit and away from home. They need time to settle in and to make friends. Many children start to work on their parents' weaknesses the moment they arrive in the unit. They tell their parents that the staff are horrible to them, that the other children don't like them or bully them and that the food is disgusting. They say that no one ever gets better in the unit, that all the children are far more ill than they are and thus the unit is not right for them. They often say that all the other children are very negative and try to avoid food, quite unlike her who has now seen the light, loves eating, wants to get better and is only being dragged down by being in a unit with such ill people. If you leave her in the unit she promises she will only get worse. She will tell you that she will now eat at home and put on her weight without any problem. She will point out that you could take her home and see and always bring her back if she does not eat as promised. However, I have never seen a child discharged from our unit against medical advice go home and eat her way to a healthy weight. They sometimes eat for a week, maybe two, but they soon feel they are alone and unsupported and they slip back into their old ways. I once remember a case of a mother who gave in to her pleading daughter and discharged her against our advice. Three hours after arriving home, her daughter took 60 paracetamol and was admitted to the intensive care unit at her local hospital. She pushed her mother to take her home but deep down she wanted her mother to be firm and support her in the difficult task of getting better. Once she realized her mother was unable to help her she panicked.

Working with the 'experts'

One thing has become very clear to us over the years and that is the enormous role that parents play in the fight for recovery. We are now quite expert at identifying those parents who will be our allies in the battle and those who despite our best efforts collude with their child's illness and cannot bring themselves to fight alongside us. We understand the difficulty. Unless you can be sure that your child is separate from her illness, and realize that when you make difficult decisions you are making a stand against her anorexia and not against your child, you are lost.

Children do not ask to develop anorexia and even those who deny they have a problem or who state clearly that they do not want to get better still need your help. Many parents, seeing the distress that it causes their child to make them eat, decide that it is kinder to give in and keep their daughter happy. This happiness is very short lived. Children do not want to be left alone with their anorexia and parents who cannot be tough are in effect abandoning their child to the whims of the illness. We often speak to parents whose child is in desperate need of in-patient treatment. We sometimes spend hours trying to persuade these parents that they have to make this difficult decision themselves. It is quite unfair of them to ask a very sick child whether or not they want treatment. Children have the right to expect their older and wiser parents to make the right decision for them.

We often give the example of a child with leukaemia needing painful and unpleasant treatment. Very few parents would dream of refusing treatment on the grounds that their sick 14-year-old did not want it. Why, we often ask ourselves, are parents so often content to leave their child completely alone to struggle with an equally life-threatening disease. Throughout this book we constantly remind you that your child's anorexia can be overcome if you are prepared to fight it alongside the professionals. One child and her illness cannot win against such a team of adults, but if you leave your child unsupported and allow her illness to drive a wedge between you and her doctors, you might be allowing it to take over her life for many years to come.

It makes me angry when parents say, 'Its up to her, she's old enough to make her own decisions.' She might be old enough but she certainly isn't well enough. I've even heard a parent say of her 13-year-old 'I agree with you doctor, I've told her she's going to die.' If you want your child to get better, and more importantly to stay better, you must be prepared for a very long, hard battle, a battle to save her life.

Having identified anorexia as the enemy to overcome, you need to know what will happen if you do nothing as the long-term outlook for someone with untreated anorexia is bleak.

If your child tells you horror stories about what is going on in the unit, do discuss it with the staff before you make decisions. You will probably find that things have been wildly exaggerated or twisted a little.

Also check with staff before you act on instructions that your child has passed onto you. Remember that the children who were once honest and truthful become more than a little devious once in the grip of anorexia nervosa.

It is not helpful to the unit if you try to negotiate your child's target weight down. The weight set is the minimum one at which she will be healthy. Cutting it will mean that she does not reach puberty or regain her periods. Your child will never be happy with her target weight until she is completely cured, as however far you try to lower it, it would never be low enough for her. Don't fall for the old plea that if only you would allow her to be 2kg under her target weight she would happily stay at the unit, they never do. Two kilograms become 3, becomes 4, 5 and 6kg below target weight very quickly.

Tough choices

Another major problem we encounter in our unit is from parents who promise to discharge their daughter either just before the end of the programme or after three to four weeks. They want the unit to persuade her to eat but they think that once she has been eating for three to four weeks she would continue to do so at home. In some cases the parents never intend to discharge their child early, but think this is a good way of settling her in. In fact, it is the worst thing they can do. If a child believes that she is to be discharged in three to four weeks, or if she believes that her parents will discharge her if she convinces them that the unit is not helping her, she has no incentive at all to settle in and form relationships with staff who could help her overcome her illness. A child who is marking time or is intent on providing evidence that the unit is useless, is obviously going to make sure that this is indeed the case. It is a waste of her time making any investment at all in the unit or its therapy because she will soon be gone, or so she hopes.

What often happens is that, after three or four weeks, parents realize that their child is not really ready for discharge and tell her that they've changed their minds and she is staying. The sudden disappointment usually precipitates some sort of crisis such as taking an overdose or running away. She feels very let down. It is much better to be honest from the outset. Tell your child that she is staying in the unit until the doctors decide that she is well enough to go home rather than taking the risk that you may have to dash her hopes at a later stage.

If you are able to support the unit and the work they are doing, your child will be better able to accept the help. If you are negative about the programme, she will feel justified in rubbishing everything there is on offer.

If your child refuses to eat in the unit, it may be that the staff have no choice but to feed her through a naso-gastric tube. It is something we do very rarely in our clinic. It happens only once every one or two years that we are sent a child who will not eat for us. When it happens, it is a very serious situation. It is not possible to sit back and watch a child, who has been admitted because of grave concerns over her physical health, continue to starve herself. On the very rare occasions that this happens, I have no qualms at all about passing a naso-gastric tube and feeding the child. I am responsible for her and I would be failing in my duties both to her and her parents if I left her without food. If a patient at Rhodes Farm refuses her very first meal she would be fed – we don't give them any chances, there is no negotiation, they have to eat. Passing a naso-gastric tube is often referred to as force-feeding. I think it is quite wrong to describe it in this way. It is a non-traumatic, very quick procedure and force is very seldom necessary. Most children sit quietly while the tube is passed and co-operate with the procedure.

The tube is about the thickness of a ballpoint pen refill and is made of very soft flexible rubber. It does not hurt and passing the tube causes no harm at all. Once the tube has been threaded through the nose and into the stomach, it is attached with a piece of tape, and milk or other liquid foods can be syringed down the tube and into the stomach. At Rhodes Farm we remove the tube after each meal rather than assume that a child will still refuse to eat the next meal. If she does refuse the next meal we pass it again. In most cases children give up their fight and eat after having had one meal through the tube as they see the futility of what they are doing. At Rhodes Farm the children are told that there are two ways to go. The easy way which is to eat, put on weight and take part in all the activities, and the hard way which is to be fed via a tube. Either way the child puts on weight so her struggling makes no difference to the outcome. Most parents support our very clear message that whichever way they choose every child in Rhodes Farm gains 1kg per week.

Non co-operation

Very occasionally we have had children who have been fed via a naso-gastric tube and still have not managed to gain weight. This is a worrying situation as there are very few options left if tube feeding fails. The most common reason for not gaining weight even though the food intake is sufficient, is exercising. In units which do not specialise in the care of anorexic children, staff are often not aware of just how many calories a dedicated exerciser can work off. Twenty-four-hour supervision is the only way to combat this problem.

Vomiting is another way that a child may avoid putting on weight whilst being fed. Usually the tube is regurgitated when the child vomits and the nurses are immediately aware of what has happened. However, some tubes have weighted ends and stay in the stomach even after vomiting. Total supervision, especially on trips to the toilet or shower, will stop any vomiting.

A more devious away to counter the effects of tube feeding is to steal a syringe and draw the liquid back up the tube and shoot it into flower vases, cups or out of windows.

One last way which is often over-looked is the problem with food absorption. We have found that some children who are being tube fed have a problem with digesting and absorbing the milky liquid we put down the tube. We have seen children go to the toilet and pass the white milk out almost unchanged. We think this has something to do with the fact that we are feeding them continuously instead of at intervals as proper meals would be. We suspect that they cannot make enough of the enzymes necessary to aid digestion. We get over this by using a mixture which contains very little dairy produce, a mixture of vegetable cream and smooth peanut butter and give it six times a day instead of continuously.

Instead of tube feeding a very difficult patient, some units have another system of introducing food into the stomach. They insert a permanent tube directly through the body and through the stomach which is something that needs doing in an operating theatre and under anaesthetic. I have never understood why such a procedure needs to be undertaken when a naso-gastric tube serves the same purpose with no scarring and a fraction of the risk. To my mind it is not something that should ever be done to someone suffering from anorexia nervosa.

Whilst there are some clinicians carrying out heroic interventions such as permanent stomach tubes, there are others who seem to do very little. I have heard cases of teenagers being sent home from units where they have refused to eat because 'they are not co-operating with the programme'.

If an anorexic co-operated with the programme, she would not need to be in a unit. This non co-operation is the very basis of her life-threatening illness. I cannot begin to imagine how the parents of a starving child must feel when she is sent home from a unit for not eating. If this should happen, you need to marshal the help of your MP, solicitor or local newspaper. There are units where even the most difficult of patients are fed successfully and you must make sure that your child is sent to one of them.

Similarly, I have heard of teenagers who have been admitted to hospital and put on saline drips, i.e. given only fluids and no calories. The staff make no attempt to feed them and seem to think that they have the right to die if they wish. When I think of how hard some doctors fight to keep alive children who have physical illnesses such as cancer I can never understand why some clinicians are not prepared to fight a little more to save someone who is clearly not thinking rationally and whose only obstacle to living a normal happy life is depression, probably caused by the malnutrition he or she could correct very easily.

You may have to be prepared to fight and struggle for your child's life. Don't be put off. In some areas it is the people who shout the loudest and protest the most who get the best treatment for their children.

Parents' support group

Some units run a support group for parents. These groups can be extremely useful especially for parents whose children have just been admitted. They find it reassuring to discuss their problems with other parents and find that they experienced similar problems with their children. It is easy to feel alone and desperate about an anorexic child's behaviour and such a relief to know that they will come through it and get better.

If your unit doesn't run a support group, you could ask for the telephone numbers of parents whose children are at the same stage as your daughter or have recovered. There are usually parents who are happy to help in this way. Some parents get together and organise their own support group, and most units will encourage you if you want to do this.

COMING HOME AGAIN

At some point in the programme you will be asked to take your child home, or to a restaurant, and you will once again be responsible for her eating. This is a big step for a child who has been eating in a unit and it is very important that you begin as you mean to continue. The staff will tell you how much your child should eat. In many cases children want to test their parents to see what they can get away with. They will be wondering whether you are stronger, more united and better placed since your family meetings to battle with her illness or if you could be persuaded to collude with her.

Your child is unlikely to be cured of her anorexia even though she has spent a long time in a unit. She should be making progress and on the right track but will need your continuing support and vigilance. Don't be persuaded to turn a blind eye to any tricks or to let her leave a bit of food you really know she should eat. It is only storing up trouble for you later. A little bit of food left today will be even more left tomorrow and in the end you will have the battle that you should have had on day one.

Above all, don't be tempted to mislead the nurses about what she has eaten. Children quite often drop their parents in it by telling the nurses that they didn't actually eat as much as their parents said. In exactly the same way, if you are not keeping a close eye on your child and she manages to offload part of her meal, she will probably boast to friends and maybe nurses to about how she has managed to hoodwink you.

You can help the nurses in their task by reporting faithfully how your child has behaved, even if it shows her in a bad light.

We all understand how difficult teenagers can be and when they are unwell the problems are exacerbated. I think parents sometimes feel that they have let their children down in some way because they have had to be admitted to a unit. They then think that they have to make amends or their child won't like them anymore. By now you should realize that the very best way you can help your child recover is to stand firm. Think long term – only by finally recovering from her eating disorder will your child be in a position to return your love and care properly.

Living with an anorexic child

Whether your child has just been diagnosed or has already had a spell in a specialist unit, living with her will now involve a knowledge of food and nutrition to enable you to support her properly and help her recover.

ESSENTIAL FOOD FACTS

The most important thing you can do now is to ensure that your child gains weight. This may not be as easy as it sounds. First you will need to know these essential food facts.

Calories

You need to know a few of the facts about so-called 'healthy eating' and make a concerted effort to match what is usually an extraordinary knowledge of calorific values. Although most children who become anorexic can recite a calorie book, there are a minority of these children who are sensible enough to realize that they are eating so little that calories are unimportant. So many parents tell us that their child appears to eat really well. This is usually either because they see her eat the odd chocolate bar, not realizing this is all she eats, or that she eats massive plates of vegetables which contain virtually no calories.

Having mastered the art of calorie counting you can move on to understanding a little about metabolism and the myths of so-called 'healthy eating'. In the next few chapters I will arm you with the facts you need to counter all your daughter's objections to eating a normal teenage diet. If you know just a little about basic nutrition you will be streets ahead of your child, who probably relies on teenage magazines for her information. Be aware that although most children who suffer from anorexia nervosa do not binge and vomit, they might turn to vomiting as a way of dealing with your new-found insistence that she eats. Likewise she may mistakenly believe that she can combat what she sees as an excess of food by taking vast quantities of laxatives. Be vigilant – both these problems are much easier to deal with if they are picked up early.

The extra calories you encourage your anorexic child to eat will initially be used to repair her damaged muscles and in order to do this it is essential that she eats plenty of protein in her diet. Over-eating 1,000 calories a day on a regular basis might be appealing to some of us but to most anorexic children it is a nightmare they will do anything to avoid. Being able and willing to count calories accurately will mean that you can control your child's weight gain very precisely and avoid her making massive gains which will frighten her, or losing precious grams which will frighten you.

Arm yourself with a good calorie book, but not one that tells you about the calories in branded foods as these are unnecessarily complicated. If you buy tinned foods or fresh chilled meals from shops like Marks and Spencer, the calories will almost always be clearly marked on the packet. Do be careful to distinguish between the numbers of calories in the whole pot or packet and the number of calories in 100g of the product. Don't mix up the kilojoules with the kilocalories, the kilojoules are always the smaller number. When you are cooking your own meals you will need to work out how many grams of butter, flour, rice, etc. you are using so that you can calculate how many calories you have put into the entire dish. You will then have to estimate what proportion of the dish your daughter will eat. When you are cooking, estimating calories is a time-consuming process. Keep a note of the calories each time so that when you repeat the recipe you don't have to recalculate. You will learn quickly the calorific values of food you use often such as butter, cheese and cream. Round the calories down and not up, and if in doubt underestimate rather than overestimate. Don't let your child be party to your calculations and don't let her interfere with your weighing and measuring. It will cause rows and disagreements which are best avoided. Keep her out of the kitchen and remember that you are in charge, not her.

At Rhodes Farm we rely very heavily on supermarket pre-prepared chilled individual meals. The calories are clearly marked on the packages and therefore avoid arguments. We often bump up the calories by sprinkling grated cheese on the top, adding butter to the sauce etc. You will find some helpful, calorie-laden recipes in Appendix 1.

A calorie is a unit of energy, simply a measurement of the amount of heat given off when we burn a certain food. Any calories consumed over and above those needed for sustaining exercise, growth, keeping warm and repairing damaged muscles are used to make fat reserves which are stored under the skin. These fat reserves are normal and indeed vital for the everyday functioning of our bodies.

Whatever your anorexic daughter tells you, be assured that a calorie is a calorie no matter what sort of food it comes from. The body has no way of telling, nor any need to tell, whether it comes from apples or butter. What counts in gaining or losing weight is the total number of calories from any source, consumed in a day or a week.

Metabolic rate

Even when asleep or completely resting, the body uses up calories. The calories are burnt to provide energy for breathing, keeping the body warm, the heart beating and thinking. About 60–70 per cent of all calories consumed are used in this way and the rest are used for extra activities. The number of calories that a person uses up when resting varies from person to person and is a function of how much muscle that person has. Growing children have a proportionally higher metabolic rate than adults. The number of calories used up during activities such as sitting, standing or jogging is also related to the metabolic rate. The higher the rate, the more calories are consumed for a given amount of exercise.

During starvation, muscle is lost from the body as well as fat and the metabolic rate is lowered. Without sufficient food to provide energy, the body tries to conserve energy by cutting down on non-essential functions. Hair, nails and skin all suffer.

They become dry and hair fails to grow. Children who are starving no longer grow in height. The thyroid gland, which controls metabolic rate, ceases to function normally, resulting in a low body temperature and constipation. The heart beats much slower than normal during starvation, a worrying sign in children that must be closely monitored. The lethargy and depression that accompany starvation are probably also protective mechanisms to ensure that no more energy is used up than is absolutely necessary. By compensating in this way, the body is able to adapt to a lower intake of food, the result is a damaged body and a very poor quality of life.

Similarly, people who repeatedly go on very low-calorie diets or skip meals lose an increased proportion of their weight as muscle and end up adapting to their poor food intake by lowering their metabolic rate. This obviously has the effect of making further weight loss more difficult and the dieter is caught in a vicious circle.

When an anorexic child is eating sufficient food to increase her weight, the opposite happens. The metabolic rate rises in line with the increased intake of food and even after reaching target weight and dropping her calories to a maintenance level, her metabolic rate may remain high for several months. If this is the case, she will have to eat more food than is normal simply to keep her weight stable.

As we have already discussed, the energy we need to grow and move comes from the food we eat. Food provides us with carbohydrates, fats and proteins as well as vitamins and minerals.

Carbohydrates

These provide the body with energy and can be converted into body fat if eaten in excess. Carbohydrates can be divided into sugars and starches. The main sources of sugars in the diet are of course sugar, soft drinks, fruit juice, cakes, biscuits and sweets. Starches are typically found in potatoes, cereals and flour.

One gram of carbohydrate gives us 4 calories. It is recommended that we eat about 50 per cent of our calories as carbohydrates. For many teenagers, carbohydrates are the most significant part of their diet. Carbohydrates release energy quickly and so provide immediate energy for children who need to be keeping their energy levels high. Normal children sometimes eat as much as 60 per cent of their diet as carbohydrates.

Proteins

Proteins are used for growth and repair and can also be used for energy. Proteins are made up of compounds called amino acids. Amino acids are divided into two groups, essential amino acids which cannot be made by the body and can only be obtained from food and non-essential ones which are equally essential but can be made by the body using other amino acids in the diet.

Protein can come from animal or vegetable sources. Vegetable proteins come from food such as lentils, beans and nuts. Animal proteins come from meat, fish, cheese, milk and eggs.

Protein cannot be stored so we need to supply the body with an assortment of different proteins every day. Like carbohydrates, proteins provide 4 calories of energy per gram and teenagers need at least 50gm of protein a day. In children who are regaining weight and have damaged their muscles through starvation, 20 per cent of their calories each day must be protein. If the body does not have a large enough supply of carbohydrate or fats, it will use protein as energy in preference to using it for growth and repair.

Fats

Fats are a more concentrated form of energy than carbohydrates. They provide twice as many calories per gram as carbohydrates, i.e. 9 calories. Despite the bad press given to fats, they are an essential part of our diet and children should not have less than 30 per cent of their daily calories as fat. As a nation we currently eat about 40 per cent of our diet as fat. Fats are divided into saturated and unsaturated fats. In general, saturated fats are solid at room temperature, like butter and lard, and unsaturated fats tend to be liquid, such as fish oil and olive oil. Foods containing fat provide us with very important fat-soluble vitamins, E, A, D and K. Fat also releases its energy more slowly than carbohydrates and so helps to stabilise the appetite between meals.

There is a lot of controversy about which fats are good for us and which should be avoided. Some fats are actually protective. Articles about weight, heart disease and dietary guidelines are making us obsessed with low-fat diets. It does seem as though we should try to cut down on processed fats, such as margarine, and fats that have been heated to fry or deep-fry foods. What we most definitely need are essential fatty acids which are actually beneficial to our health. They can increase metabolism, protect the heart and increase memory and concentration. These essential fats are present in oily fish, nuts, corn oil and sunflower oil, but remember they are damaged by heats so they should not be heated strongly. We can eat animal fats such as butter, cheese, cream, and fats found in meat in moderation, and we certainly should not worry about how much fat our children eat. Many growing children need as many as 4,000 calories a day and if they were to try and take these in as carbohydrates they would have great difficulties. As fats provide energy in a more concentrated form, children may well need a higher percentage of their diet as fat. Children who are being re-fed certainly come into this category. High-fat foods are lower in bulk and are easier to eat than high carbohydrate food. One interesting point is that whilst many anorexic children will tell you that they are avoiding fat because they are worried about their heart, they are not aware that during periods of starvation, blood cholesterol rises to very high levels, much higher than would be seen in a normal child. In their defence, I have to say that I can understand why many children develop a fat phobia – they are constantly bombarded with advice about following low-fat diets. It certainly does not make sense that these children risk heart failure, kidney damage, bone problems and infertility in the mistaken belief that they are avoiding blocked heart arteries. We often point out to them that what we see before us is certainly not a picture of health and they would have done better to have eaten hamburgers and chips non-stop.

Milk in another cause for concern amongst most anorexics. They almost all want to drink skimmed milk instead of the extremely nutritious whole milk which is unprocessed and as nature intended. The difference in calories between skimmed milk and whole milk is ridiculously small and yet anorexics will vigorously argue their right to drink skimmed milk. The average saving on a bowl of cereal is 40 calories. There is some evidence to suggest that a lack of fat in the diet might be responsible for the depression which often accompanies anorexia. Other researchers have suggested that a low-fat diet might contribute to the feelings which make people indulge in self-harm. We somehow need to make children realize that fat does not make you fat, too many calories make you fat.

By far the majority of children admitted to our clinic claim to be vegetarian. Most of their parents will explain that their sudden concern about the welfare of animals coincided with or just predates the beginning of their illness. It is very difficult to produce a diet high in good quality protein sufficient for the needs of a child without using meat and fish.

At Rhodes Farm we insist that the children eat fish and chicken breast although we do not insist on them eating red meat. This rule is a good one for parents to follow, especially parents of anorexic children who will not be prepared to eat milk, eggs, cream and cheese in the large quantities necessary if they are to provide the only source of animal protein. Unfortunately, most children who say that they are going to become vegetarians eat only vegetables. They make little or no attempt to replace the protein lost by not eating meat. Children who eat vegan diets do not thrive. Asian children who eat like this are often very anaemic, they tend to be tired at school and do not excel at games and sports. Fish and chicken are excellent sources of first class protein, they have little fat content and therefore not too many calories. Vegetarianism should be reserved for adults who have finished their growing and can hopefully make sensible decisions about how to replace the lost protein. We see a remarkable number of vegetarian children who do not like vegetables!

Fibre

Fibre is another concern among anorexic children. We read endlessly about the need to eat plenty of fibre in our diet. Most children eating a mixed and varied diet consume sufficient fibre without having to worry about eating certain foods. Brown bread, for example, should be eaten because one prefers the taste not simply for the small amount of fibre it contains. It is usually accepted that brown bread is 'better' than white bread but in fact white bread contains more vitamins and minerals. Few teenagers realize that if we eat too much fibre it prevents the absorption of calcium, vital for healthy teeth and bones.

DAILY PLAN

Begin by telling your child (not asking her) what you propose to do. Explain that the rules have now changed; from now on, she eats what you ask her to eat, when you ask her to eat and she eats with the family, never alone.

Weighing and measuring

Weighing an anorexic child is not as simple as it sounds. Children discover early on in their treatment that the weight they are asked to reach is directly related to their height. It is therefore obvious that all except the very young and naïve will do their best to take a centimetre or two off their height. Experimentation will demonstrate how easy this is to do. Without bending one's knees, which is an obvious ploy, one can drop one's shoulders and reduce one's height by about two centimetres. Accurate measuring is best done at a clinic or GP surgery using fixed height measures. Someone needs to see that heels, bottom, shoulders and head are all firmly touching the wall before the height is read. When a child has stunted her growth through starvation, refeeding can cause a very large growth spurt. For this reason, young children need to be measured every two to three months so that adjustments can be made to their target weight.

Doctors and nurses, as well as parents, are often guilty of inaccurate weighing. When we are concerned about a child's weight, small changes in either direction are important clues as to whether we are winning or losing the battle. It is therefore vital that when we weigh every three to four days or every week that we are comparing like with like. The most accurate weight and one which we insist upon for our patients is an early morning weight. This is a weight recorded before someone has eaten or drunk but after they have been to the toilet. We weigh our patients in their pants, or bra and pants on, but with no other clothing or jewellery. All too often, we hear about children who have been weighed by nurses in their clothes, often including their Doc Martens which weigh at least 1kg. You need to appreciate how vital it is to some of these children to appear to have gained a few hundred grams. It is often the basis for a decision about whether or not the child can continue at school or indeed at home. It is extremely easy for any child weighed in anything more than bra and pants to hide batteries, bags of 1p coins or similar heavy articles in pockets or under baggy T-shirts. A current favourite is to buy wrist and ankle weights designed for body builders and push them high under T-shirt sleeves, or tie them with string around the waist. They weigh about 1kg each and three or four of them are easy to lose under even light clothing. A wide hairband can also secrete six to eight large batteries, especially under long hair. Heavy metal bangles and pendants can also add much-needed grams when the chips are down. These tricks are relatively easy to spot once one knows what to look for, but less easy to police is water drinking. One litre of fluid weighs 1kg and anyone can artificially boost their weight temporarily by drinking just before they are weighed. At our clinic we do a weekly reconnaissance, checking rooms, cisterns and behind bath panels for bottles of water, measuring jugs and illicit bathroom scales. Despite warnings from us, parents find out the hard way how devious their children can be. Children can train themselves to drink more and more water. It is a very dangerous pursuit but these very sick children ignore the risks. When someone drinks 3, 4 or 5 litres of fluid in a short space of time, the body fluids become diluted and this causes the brain to swell. As the brain is inside a completely rigid skull, it becomes crushed and damaged, causing epileptic fits and blindness. We had a patient at the clinic who drank 5 litres of water one day to disguise weight loss and spent the next few days fighting for her life in an intensive care unit. Her eye-sight was permanently damaged.

Many parents tell us that they know they have an accurate weight because they woke their child and weighed her immediately. They are unaware that these children set their alarm for 3 or 4 o'clock in the morning and tank up early, and some even train themselves to drink the night before and to sleep with an extremely full bladder. You will not hear them go to the bathroom as the water is usually hidden in litre bottles in their rooms. There is only one sure way to detect water drinking and that is to spot weigh your child at least once a week. This means you suddenly announce your intention to weigh her at a time when she is least expecting it. You should do it at completely random times, an hour or two after her weekly weighing, one day as she walks in from school, just before bed, midday at the weekend. It is almost impossible for someone to over drink any significant amount on a full-time basis as it is usually only held for an hour or two. It is important that there is an element of surprise for a spot weight to be useful; we have heard of children who drink water every day before leaving school because their parents regularly spot check them at this time. If your child knows that she will be spot checked at least every week, you will relieve her of the responsibility of having to decide whether or not to drink water. You are helping to keep her safe, for it is very unlikely that she will do it knowing that she is certain to be caught out.

If you do not feel able to insist on weighing your child in her underwear, you will have to arrange for her to be weighed at your GP's surgery.

It is wise to mention tactfully that you would like her weighed in her bra and pants. If your child is being weighed by her GP, you will still need to spot check her. If you do this, you must remember that she should weigh approximately ½ - 1kg more during the day than she would first thing in the morning. Also, allow about a kilogram for the weight of her clothes. Finally, remember a spot check is never accurate; you are only trying to pick up large changes caused by water drinking.

If you have a child who has lost or is losing weight and you want to help her reach a healthy weight, it is vital to have a thorough understanding of calories. In order to gain 1kg a week one has to over eat 7,000 calories, i.e. 1,000 calories a day over and above what is needed to stay stable. The average child needs between 1,500 and 2,500 kcal a day in order to maintain her weight. These calories are used to provide the energy for growth, keeping warm and moving around. The exact number of kilocalories needed will depend on how active your child is. If she is driven to school and comes home and reads books or watches television, 1,500 calories may suffice. If however she cycles, swims, is in the school team for sports and likes to walk the dog, she will need 2,500 calories a day or even more. To gain 1kg a week her daily allowance needs to rise to between 2,500 and 3,500 kilocalories.

Anorexics who feel guilty and disgusted with themselves for eating a Mars bar should realize that even if it provided over and above the calories they needed every day for maintenance, a 300kcal chocolate bar would only put on 40g (or just over 1 ounce) in weight. They would need to eat 23 on top of their normal daily intake to gain 1kg. Most normal people avoid putting on weight simply by eating the correct number of calories needed each day. They do this automatically without having to count calories or consult packets.

You will need to count calories fairly accurately in order to follow this scheme, so a calorie book is vital. Your daughter will probably know more about calories than the person who wrote the calorie book but nevertheless do not be persuaded to take her word on the calorific value of any foods. Make your own 'guesstimates' of the values of food you cook, always erring on the side of caution, and round everything down not up as your daughter will doubtless be doing. Do not allow her to be involved in shopping or food preparation. It is quite normal for teenagers to eat what they are given, and in fact very few of them hang around the kitchen to see how much butter goes into the mashed potato.

Your child should begin by eating 1,500 kcal a day for the first three days. This is less than a healthy child eats to maintain her weight and cannot be considered a large amount of food. This should be eaten as three 500-kcal meals. The meals should consist of normal food. Bread must be buttered, cereals must have milk on them and the meals should be exactly the kind other teenagers eat. Do not avoid creamy sauces, cheese, chips or pastry. Remember that your child has to gain weight, you and the rest of your family do not. Do not be tempted to eat to keep her company or to insist that your other children eat desserts when they are not in the habit of doing so. Anorexic children often love to prepare recipes laden with butter and cream for their parents and siblings to eat. It helps them feel in control if they can resist eating them. It also stems from their need to nurture others. Do be on the look-out for any sign that she is pressurising her brothers or sisters to overeat. It is a common occurrence and one which needs to be stopped. Explain to your child that over the next few weeks she has to eat more to make up for all the food she has missed.

Butter, cream, cheese and chocolate are not bad foods. Because of their high calories, using them to help weight gain has the advantage of lowering the bulk of food that the child has to eat. A 500-kcal portion of fish and chips or chicken korma and rice is tiny in comparison with a 500-kcal meal of grilled chicken breast with boiled potatoes or pasta and tomato sauce. A normal teenage diet should contain not less than 30 per cent fat, and increasing this in the short term to help someone gain weight will not harm their health or increase their risk of coronary heart disease, but it will make their meals easier to cope with.

For the first seven days follow the calorie programme as follows:

Day 1	1,500 kcal
Day 2	1,500 kcal
Day 3	1,500 kcal
Day 4	2,000 kcal
Day 5	2,000 kcal
Day 6	2,500 kcal
Day 7	2,500 kcal

Weigh your child before you begin the calorie programme but do not weigh her again during the first week and lock up your scales so that she cannot weigh herself. Explain to her that during this first week, she could appear to gain 2 or even 3kg. This is not real weight; she will not look any different because it is simply the effect of filling her intestine with waste food and readjusting her water balance. This disproportionate weight gain in the first week is a one-off effect which will not be repeated. You must prepare her so that she will not panic when you weigh her on Day 8. Reassure her that after the first week you will adjust her calories every three to four days to make sure she does not gain more than 1kg a week. Weigh your child on Day 8. This must be a weight recorded first thing in the morning, before she has eaten or drunk but after she has been to the toilet. She must be weighed in her bra and knickers or a swimming costume.

Create a graph like on page 120 and mark this Day 8 weight on the bottom of the graph. Fill in the rest of the weights on the graph every three to four days all the way to her target weight. Continue to see that your child eats 2,500 kcal a day and weigh her again on Day 11. You will now have to adjust her calories according to her weight gain. If she is on the line, you do nothing and she continues to eat the same calories each day. If she is one square below the line, you must increase her calories by 250 a day. If she is two squares below the line, you must increase her calories by 500 a day. If she is one square above the line, you must cut her calories by 250 a day. If she is two squares above the line, you must cut her calories by 500 a day. Continue to weigh her every three to four days and adjust her calories each time to ensure her weight stays as close to the line as possible. You must stop all exercise, even walking, all the time that her weight is the line. She may do one piece of exercise a day once her weight is over 75 per cent of the target weight and as long as her weight is above the line. If you stick rigidly to this rule, she will be extremely motivated to gain her kilogram each week and to make up any weight if she falls behind.

If your child remains one to two squares below the line, even though you increased her calories three or four days before, her calories must be increased again in exactly the same way. If your child does not gain weight eating 3,500 kcal a day, she is most certainly cheating in some way. The first reason for someone not to gain weight eating 3,500 kcal a day is that they are not in fact eating this much food, but simply leading you to believe that they are. You must count her calories accurately. Do not be tempted to think that she is eating enough as she is eating a large volume of food. It is possible to eat a lot of food such as fruit and vegetables which have very little energy value at all, without gaining weight. Be aware that plates of carrots, sprouts, pasta, baked potatoes, fruit, dry cereal and diet yoghurts contain few, if any, calories and eating them in order to gain weight is a waste of time.

You can only believe the food that you see your daughter eat, not the empty wrappers or the swearing on the Bible, nor the fact that the food has disappeared. You cannot afford to turn your back for one second, as this is all it takes to magic a chocolate bar under the cushion, into a tissue or under a hair band.

Check that the milk has not been watered down or that cereals have not had the nuts removed or indeed the packet filled with bran. Inspect the contents of the Mars bar wrapper. It may conceal a low-calorie chocolate bar, not a Mars bar at all.

Put butter on bread and toast yourself, and watch to see that it isn't squeezed into sleeves, serviettes or tissues or smeared under the table. Watch that food doesn't miraculously jump from the plate onto someone else's plate or onto the floor.

Another favourite trick is to blow one's nose throughout the meal, each time spitting mouthfuls of food into the tissue. Children who do this come to the table with sleeves packed with paper tissues. Chocolate bars and desserts can also be expertly packed into the cheeks and as long as one is not asked to speak one can escape the table and spit it out.

You will easily spot a child who hides food in her clothes. They are stained and greasy with remnants if food left in the pockets. Food that is smuggled from the table is often left hidden in the bedroom in bags, in cupboards, left to rot, smell and be discovered. In most cases leaving the food where it is sure to be found is a clear cry for help and parents should respond by searching the child before she leaves the table and regularly check her bedroom. This is not an intrusion of privacy, it is simply responding to a non-verbal request for someone to care enough to stop her. Ignoring these signals is cruelty not kindness.

Other reasons that someone might eat 3,500 kcal and not gain weight is because they are seriously over-exercising or they are vomiting. Both these problems are fully dealt with in other chapters. We have never seen someone genuinely eat 3,500 kcal and not gain weight who isn't exercising or vomiting.

Remember to spot check your daughter's weight randomly once a week to ensure that she is not drinking water to boost her weight artificially. As your child gets closer to target weight, her metabolism will increase and she will have to eat an increasingly large amount in order to gain 1kg a week.

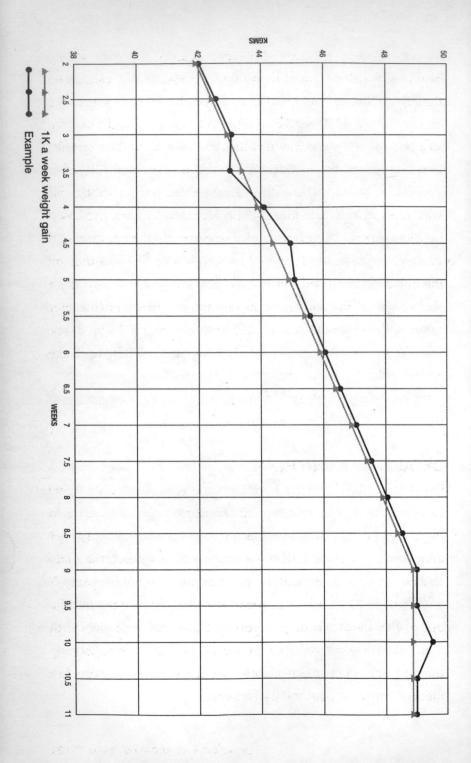

KGMS

50

48

46

44

42

40

38

2 2.5 3 3.5 4 4.5 5 5.5 6 6.5 7 7.5 8 8.5 9 9.5 10 10.5 11

WEEKS

1K a week weight gain

Example

You need to the Day 8 weight against the spot at the beginning of Week 2 and then fill in the rest of the weights on the vertical line to your child's target weight. In the example, the child weighed 42kg on Day 8. She had a target weight of 49kg so a horizontal line is drawn at that line weight. In the example, the child gained ?kg to 42.5kg by Day 11 and reached 43kg after 1 week, i.e. Day 15. Three days later she still weighed 43kg and was thus one square below the line. Her calories were increased by 250 a day and all exercise was stopped. By the beginning of Week 4, she had caught up and weighed 44kg. She was thus on the line and continued to eat 2,750 kcal a day. Three days later she weighed 45kg and was thus one square above the line. Her calories were therefore cut by 250 kcal back to 2,500 kcal a day. She then continued to gain a steady kilogram in weight until she reached target weight.

It might be necessary to make more frequent adjustments than we have made in our example.

DETAILS OF MENU PLAN

On days 1, 2 and 3 children are expected to eat only 1,500 calories. This is less than a maintenance diet but it is safer to begin slowly when someone has not been used to eating. Do not allow your daughter to leave a single scrap of food; the plate must be scraped clean and the yoghurt pot emptied properly. If you allow her to mash and spread her food, or pick the middle out of her sandwich or pie, you will fuel her obsession with food. She should be eating in a relaxed way, not constantly thinking about how many calories she can save by smearing her meal or squeezing out the mayonnaise.

At our clinic, the children are given a piece of bread to wipe their plate with if they eat badly. If butter is squeezed out of toast onto the plate or hands, the muffin is re-buttered. All milk in the cereal bowl has to be finished. Clear cut rules like these absolve them from the responsibility of having to avoid a few calories and they can eat normally without feeling guilty. If you see your child eating in a way that would embarrass you if you had guests for dinner, you should stop her immediately. Many parents are so relieved to see their child eating that they are prepared to turn a blind eye to table manners and ignore even the most disgusting rituals, which is not helpful in the long term.

Breakfast

Choose one of the high-calorie muesli as they provide a lot of calories in a low volume. Look at the calories per 100 g marked on the box and calculate how much your child needs in order to provide the correct number of calories. Weigh the cereals yourself; do not allow your child to do it. Pour the milk yourself, do not drown it but put on a normal amount. Do not use skimmed milk as she is not on a diet.

The cereal should be followed by a buttered muffin or two pieces of medium sliced bread, toasted and buttered. Orange juice or any other fruit juice should not be the reduced-sugar kind. Sit with your child while she eats and do not leave her for a second. Do not allow her to go to school until she has eaten every last scrap. Do not enter into any deals or bargains as she will try to negotiate swapping buttered toast for something she can either hide more easily or eat later (hoping you will forget). See that she has emptied her mouth before she leaves the table and check pockets and sleeves for tissue if you suspect her of cheating. Any food you find must be replaced by a similar amount, erring on the side of caution as a disincentive to hide food again.

Lunch

Choose something from the suggested meals on page x and sit with your child while she eats. Be strict about the way in which she eats – remember it is part of her illness to eat in a ritualistic way, so you need to help her overcome it. Do not allow her to drink diet drinks. Children who are hungry but are afraid to eat drink large quantities of diet drinks to fill their stomach and satisfy their craving for sweet things. Water is fine if she wants to stick rigidly to her calories. If she wants to drink squash or coke, do not count it as part of her calories.

Most anorexic children have a phobia of food which contains fat and they will try to swap normal food for fat-free food such as drinks, fruit or cereal. Resist any requests to swap; you need to wean your daughter off the idea that there are good foods and bad foods. Yoghurts are almost all low fat, but make sure that you are not buying 'lite' yoghurts which are artificially sweetened. If your child is at school you will need to meet her at lunchtime or ask the school nurse to supervise her lunch. You cannot rely on her telling you the truth when she tells you she has eaten her lunch alone.

Your child will tell you that she is already one of the fattest children in her class, if not the fattest. She will tell you how unfair it is that you are insisting on her gaining weight and that no one has to eat as much as she does. While she is gaining weight, this may well be the case and she needs reminding that she has lost weight and her friends have not, that she has probably lost her periods, her friends have not. In fact 700 caloriesis not an abnormal amount for a teenager to eat at lunchtime and if her friends are eating less, they will certainly be eating crisps, drinks and chocolate later on.

Supper

Pick a main course in line with the suggestions made on page x. Your daughter can have vegetables if she wants them but as they add considerable bulk for almost zero calories, she should not eat too many. We do need to eat plenty of fresh fruit and vegetables every day, but in the short term while your child gains weight, her orange juice, fruit and a few vegetables will be sufficient. Use butter and melted cheese to bump up the calories on standard meals as they are a wonderful way of adding calories without volume, and enable the rest of the family to eat a similar meal without putting on weight.

You should be perfectly frank with your child about how many calories she is eating and not try to slip in extra butter or cream without her knowing. She must understand that she needs to eat 7,000 kcal in order to gain a mere 1kg, as she will have the idea that she puts on weight very easily. When her metabolism was at rock bottom due to her starvation, she certainly would have put on weight more easily but as she progresses, it becomes increasingly difficult to gain.

Your child may well try to tell you that she is full, bloated, in pain and cannot possibly eat another thing. She may panic you into letting her leave some by threatening to be sick. Overeating does not cause pain and we have to overeat thousands of calories before we are spontaneously sick. When we go to a restaurant we eat a three-course meal with a roll and butter, followed by a chocolate or two, and consume far in excess of 1,000 kcal, if not double that amount. Eating this quantity does not cause us to have stomach aches, nor to vomit. There is some evidence that prolonged starvation causes the stomach to empty more slowly than normal but stomachs do not shrink! If your child has this problem, it will not affect her ability to eat the meal but she may well still feel full a couple of hours after the meal when a normal person's stomach would have started to empty.

We provide people who say they feel sick with a well-positioned bucket but still insist that the meal goes on. It is extremely rare that they have need of the bucket.

When you make it clear that you are not going to allow your child to leave the table, she will usually finish with no further mention of feeling sick or bloated.

Both you and she need to understand that the food has to be eaten whether or not she is full; continued starvation is not an option, even if in the short term eating is in fact uncomfortable. The food has to be eaten either at home or in hospital but eaten it must be. It will help you to remind yourself that despite her pleas and distress, you are not asking her to do anything abnormal. You are simply asking her to eat enough food to keep herself alive, a thing that millions of people do everyday and thoroughly enjoy.

She may well be extremely angry and resentful, she may say some very hurtful things, but you know you are doing the right thing. You can be in no doubt that as parents it is your responsibility to keep your child safe and well. It is more sensible to suffer her tantrums now, knowing that she will have a normal future to look forward to, than to give into this illness and risk her justifiable resentment later when she is physically damaged by her anorexia. It does not matter that she 'doesn't like you' now, you are her parents, not her friends, so you must do what is in her best interests however painful it may be.

Snacks

At our clinic we insist that the first snack is always a chocolate bar. We do this because so many of the children in our care are frightened to eat chocolate. They are afraid that if they taste it, they will enjoy it and be unable to stop eating it. It is fair to say that most children like chocolate and one is branded as abnormal if one never ever eats it. Many of us offer gifts of chocolates to people without a thought that they may not like them.

Ignore pleas to eat anything other than chocolate. This is not just about feeding your child back up to a normal weight; it is about re-establishing an eating pattern that will allow her to join in socially with friends and peers. You will have similar battles about chips and cheese, so make sure you win these as they are important.

Make sure that the snacks vary. Anorexic children feel safe when they have established a plan of eating and would like to eat the same thing every day if allowed. You must not let this happen, as it is abnormal, obsessive and debilitating. Think about how she used to eat before she was ill and do not half-do the job. You owe it to her to help her recover totally from this illness. Allow her to choose from a range of snacks but do not buy any more until they have all been used and then buy a new selection. Be especially vigilant when your child is eating nuts as they are the easiest of foods to flick or hide. We have discovered bras, socks and knickers to be perfect places for hiding entire packets of nuts.

With very young children (13 or under), it is perfectly acceptable to exchange the 500-kcal dessert for a 250-kcal dessert and a chocolate bar, should they find 1,000 calories too much to eat at one meal. With children older than this you should insist that they eat a main course and a dessert. There are very few children who would turn down the chance to eat a meal like this and you are colluding with the idea that you are asking them to do something abnormal by eating two large courses. You can say that you understand that they will not always be eating meals this big. When we are invited to weddings or dinners, most of us manage to eat more than 1,000 kcal and actually enjoy it too! These children should not go through life thinking that 1,000 calorie meal is an impossibility without feeling sick and bloated.

Another problem you might run into is that of a child who, whilst not refusing to eat, eats so slowly that one meal runs into the snack and then onto the next meal. Eating slowly when being forced to eat against their will is the last little bit of control that these children feel they have left and they are often reluctant to relinquish it. You must set time limits for the meals and half an hour per meal is reasonable. You will have to impose sanctions if the time limit is not adhered to. If you find that meals are taking so long that you can no longer sit and supervise them, your child will have to understand that the only alternative is admission to a unit where there are staff who can sit at the table all day and all night if necessary until the food is finished. At work, nurses do not have other children to pick up from school or shopping to get, and they can devote all their time to feeding their patient if necessary.

Once your child reaches target weight, the line on her graph becomes horizontal and no longer slopes. You should continue to weigh your child twice a week and adjust her calories in exactly the same way as you did when she was gaining weight. You will find that your child will stabilise her weight by eating approximately 1,000 calories a day less than she did when she was gaining weight. This reduction in calories must be gradual and reductions made only when her weight is one square above the line.

Continue to weigh her twice a week for six weeks after she reaches target weight. After this you can weigh her just once a week.

You must continue to spot check your child once a week, even when she is at target, and still weigh her in her underwear or swimming costume. You must continue to ban all exercise if her weight ever drops below her target line. We often hear parents say that their child manages to stay at her target weight but appears to eat very little.

This is a common problem amongst what we would describe as controlled anorexics. This is a child who understands that she must maintain a safe weight but nevertheless is still extremely resistant to eating and is terrified of gaining a gram more than necessary.

Life can be lived at two levels. There is the level at which one eats the maximum amount without gaining weight and the level at which one eats the minimum of food without losing weight. The two levels can be 200–300 kcals a day apart. Eating as much as possible is what most children do automatically and with little thought to what or how much they are eating. They have lots of energy, run when they could walk, grow normally and are extremely fit. Controlled anorexic children often experiment with cutting their food intake and if this doesn't result in weight loss will cut down a little more. Each day they reduce their calories their body makes adjustments which compensates for the reduction in food. Initially, these adjustments are made in preference to weight loss but if the level of food intake continues to decline, a large weight loss inevitably follows.

Cutting down on food intake results in the child feeling constantly tired, lethargic and cold. Growth is impaired and hair, skin and nails suffer. Children who starve or eat insufficient food are usually depressed and we think this is due to a lack of cholesterol in the diet. These children move slowly, have little energy and although they may just be eating enough food not to lose weight, they function poorly. A minimum eater needs encouragement to raise their food intake slowly and to see that this will result in them feeling fitter and healthier but will not cause them to gain weight. An energetic child full of vitality burns off more calories than a cold depressed one.

Another possible explanation for the fact that your child eats very little but appears not to lose weight is that she is disguising her weight loss. This could be by hiding weights, by having tampered with your scales or by drinking water. These possible causes are all easily investigated if you are suspicious.

Sanctions

Parents often end up feeling that there is nothing they can do when their child disobeys them. It is true that for many anorexic children, the normal threats of not being allowed to see their friends or not going to the cinema are sanctions that will not worry them very much. However, given a little thought there are always things which will provide a meaningful sanction. It is also true that anorexic children are past-masters at cutting off their nose to spite their face and are probably less likely than most children to comply in order to avoid a punishment. But just because it might not work is not a reason for not trying. You have nothing to lose and it might help keep your child out of hospital.

As parents you are best placed to think about the sanctions that will be most effective in helping your child. We can suggest some obvious ones such as stopping pocket money, stopping television, removing records, cassettes or video games or banning outings, trips to theme parks, concerts, visits to friends or school trips. A child who does not eat cannot go to school and that would include not sitting exams. Children who eat slowly certainly should not be allowed to keep an adult at the table for two hours and then take off on a bike ride or swimming. Sitting alone in a bedroom for the same amount of time that one was at the table seems like a fitting punishment. Going to bed early or being sent to one's room is a useful sanction for many situations.

Many parents seem to find things very difficult when it comes to imposing sanctions. They either do not see eye to eye about the punishment and fall out when it comes to imposing it or cannot bring themselves to impose punishments that will really work because, 'she would be too upset and would not speak to us'.

We vividly remember, with two parents, struggling to think of a suitable sanction for their extremely rebellious daughter. Eventually one parent suggested cancelling a pop concert planned for the following week. The other parent however decided it could not be used as a punishment because their daughter was looking forward to it so much. You must remember that sanctions only have to be imposed if your child chooses of her own free will and in full knowledge of the outcome, to break the rules. She is able to avoid the sanctions if she wishes. In effect you are not punishing her; she is punishing herself. Whichever sanction you choose, the golden rule is to impose it firmly. It loses all usefulness if you move the goal posts or water down the punishment. Never give your child 'one last chance'.

At our clinic we find that threats to deprive the children of walks, swimming and other sporting activities work very well for those well enough to take part in them.

The contract

Onc thing that we often suggest is entering into a contract with the child, every day or every time you speak on the telephone or meet for a visit. The contract is aimed at reassuring a child who may genuinely feel worried and anxious about her weight without these worries dominating the entire day or the entire conversation. For some children talking about their weight becomes an obsession and they feel a constant urge to be reassured. The more often this is done, the faster the urge reappears. The feeling of well-being which they derive from being reassured lasts for a shorter and shorter period until they are needing to seek reassurance every few minutes.

The contract works like this. When you first see or speak to your child you explain that you understand that because she is ill, she has worries about being fat. You can add that, given the fact that she wears size 10 clothes, you find this difficult to understand. Not only do you find it difficult to understand but you and probably most of her friends and relatives are thoroughly bored with conversations about how she looks. You go on to suggest that you will listen for five minutes to her worries and thoughts about how fat she is or how fat she will become if she is in a unit for refeeding. You will reassure her once and once only about the fact that she is not and will not become fat and then the subject is taboo for the rest of the day. You may like to suggest some positive topics of conversation which you would like to pursue after this five-minute period. There obviously has to be some sanction if she reneges on the contract and continues to talk about weight. If she is in a unit you could say that she will be returned or that you will leave. If you are at home, you could simply withdraw from the activity you were proposing. Of course, having spelt out the proposed sanction you must be prepared to carry it out. Far from being hard and uncaring, exercises of this kind really helps your child get back some control. The intensely anxious feelings that these children experience are not pleasant and they are often unable to fight them without your help.

Medical treatment

Although anorexia nervosa is clearly a psychiatric illness, children who suffer from it experience many physical symptoms.

These symptoms need to be monitored closely and it is a good idea to have your child checked by a paediatrician at regular intervals. If she is losing weight or failing to gain weight then once-weekly checks are necessary. She should be weighed and have pulse and blood pressure taken. Insist that your child is weighed in her underwear so that she cannot hide objects that could enhance her weight.

A child needs to have her pulse and blood pressure checked as they are very good indicators of how her body is coping with being at a low weight. When her pulse slows and her blood pressure drops she must be taken into hospital or a unit where she can be fed. Equally, she should be examined for swollen ankles, a sign that the fine balance of chemicals in her body has been disturbed. Some doctors take regular blood samples to check blood potassium levels as they can drop dangerously low in children who vomit or take laxatives. She should also be checked to see that she is not dehydrated.

There is no place for drugs in the treatment of anorexia nervosa. These children need food, not tablets. There are people who advocate the use of iron, zinc or vitamin tablets but there is no evidence that they are useful. As soon as the child begins to eat a normal diet, all nutrients and vitamin deficiencies are corrected very quickly. Most children who are starving themselves are depressed, but prescribing antidepressant medication should be avoided. In most cases the depression lifts very quickly once the child is eating normally and has regained some weight. If your child has been at a target weight for two or three months and is still depressed, then a trial of antidepressants may be justified. Most antidepressant tablets take at least three weeks to have any effect so don't try to judge their effectiveness too early. If they do help, they should be continued for a few months but not for years.

Children who don't eat often become constipated but don't be tempted to buy your child laxatives. It is better to try to increase the fibre in her diet or to give her dried figs.

Some doctors prescribe the pill for girls who are not having periods. During the pill-free week between packets, people who take the pill have what is called 'withdrawal bleed'. It is in response to the sudden withdrawal of oestrogen and is not a period. The rationale for giving the pill is to provide external oestrogen and to try to protect the bones from osteoporosis. Unfortunately recent research shows that taking the pill does not improve the amount of calcium taken into the bones and does not improve bone density. Also it makes it impossible to see whether or not the child would have normal periods if she were not taking the pill, so it serves to confuse the situation.

Conclusion

LONG-TERM PROGNOSIS

There has been a lot of investigation but little consensus about the good and bad prognostic signs in anorexia nervosa. Every researcher seems to agree that the longer the duration of the illness and the longer the time from onset of symptoms to beginning treatment the worse the prognosis. Growing up in an environment where being slender is highly valued, as in the case of models, dancers, athletes or jockeys, is also associated with a poor prognosis.

A family where relationships are good and everyone is working together, and who seeks help early in the course of the illness, has the best chance of the child recovering. As a very rough guide, we can say that of all the children who suffer from anorexia nervosa about a third will make a fairly rapid recovery and another third will go on to recover, but may need two, three or even more years of support with their eating and therapy. Most of the final third will probably go on to become chronically ill, requiring ongoing treatment for their frequent relapses.

There are very many factors which interact to influence which of these three groups a particular child will be in. It is not usually possible to predict in advance. Whether or not we can influence the group a particular child falls into is not certain but one thing is sure, a child's best chance of recovery is to return to at a normal weight, and I am in no doubt that whilst we cannot control a child's mind and her thinking, we can and must control her weight. In this way we buy ourselves time for the therapy to work and do not end up with a child so physically damaged that she could never lead a normal life even if she were to recover from her anorexia.

Although with good treatment many people are completely cured of their eating disorder, there are others who will relapse during times of crisis. When they are upset, angry or anxious those who never learnt to express their emotions turn to food and use it as a weapon. Many children see not eating as a way of punishing the people they are angry with, without stopping to see that they are in fact punishing themselves.

It is an important part of any treatment to encourage children with eating disorders to verbalise their problems and worries instead of internalising them as they tend to do.

Dr Dora Black, an eminent child psychiatrist, once said that for many children with eating disorders, food, would always be their Achilles heel. When they faced a traumatic life event such as divorce or death, they would automatically be tempted to deal with their problems by not eating and thus losing weight. In the way that diabetes cannot be cured but can be perfectly well controlled by taking insulin, some people with eating disorders can learn to live with their eating problem and keep it under control. They might never be totally free of it, it might always be there in the background, but their life is not severely disrupted by it.

As with most illnesses, the best chance of making a full recovery is if the illness is detected early and the right treatment is given.

Recipes

RECIPES WITH CALORIE COUNT GIVEN

BREAKFAST

Example 1:

150ml glass orange juice	60 kcal
100ml whole milk	65 kcal
2 slices medium slice toast	165 kcal
10g butter	70 kcal
70gm M & S Crunchy Strawberry Cereal	340 kcal
Total:	700 kcal

Example 2:

150ml glass orange juice	60 kcal
130ml whole milk	75 kcal
50g Frosties	190 kcal
1 Waitrose pain au chocolate	380 kcal
Total:	705 kcal

Example 3:

150ml glass orange juice	60 kcal
100ml whole milk	65 kcal
80g Jordans Luxury Raisin Country Crisp	325 kcal

1 white muffin toasted	180 kcal
10g butter	70 kcal
Total:	700 kcal

You can chop and change these three example breakfasts to give your child some variety. Try to see that she doesn't eat the same thing every day.

OTHER HIGH CALORIE SUGGESTIONS:

Nesquik Cereal	394 kcal per 100g
Crunchy Nut Cornflakes	395 kcal per 100g
Frosties	380 kcal per 100g
Waitrose Oat Crunchy honey / raisin/ almond	425 kcal per 100g
Waitrose Maple/Pecan Crisp	461 kcal per 100g
M & S Strawberry Crunch	460 kcal per 100g
M & S Tropical Fruit Muesli	440 kcal per 100g
Jordans Four Nut Combo Country Crisp	490 kcal per 100g

Instead of toast or muffins you could give your child one of the following and adjust the calories as necessary.

M & S bagel	237 kcal each
M & S 2 x mini chocolate muffins	131 kcal each
Tesco all butter croissant	221 kcal each
Tesco pain au raisin	286 kcal each
M & S Yum Yum	296 kcal each

You do not need to give your child orange juice every day – here are some other ideas:

M & S Apple and Mango Juice (150ml glass)	*82 kcal*
Ribena 30ml concentrate & 150ml water	
79 kcal	

MID MORNING SNACK
250 kcal milk shake

200ml full cream milk	*130 kcal*
30g Häagen Daz or Tesco Finest	
Vanilla Ice Cream	*70 kcal*
1 tbs Nesquik powder	*50 kcal*

You can use other flavour Häagen Daz ice creams such as Belgian chocolate or strawberry. You will have to add a little more ice cream if you are leaving out the Nesquik.

If you haven't any high-calorie ice cream, you can use a lower one such as Iceland Vanilla, which has only 42 kcal per 28g instead of 70 kcal in Häagen Daz. You should then use twice as much ice cream or add a tablespoon of single cream.

OTHER USEFUL MID-MORNING SNACKS
Biscuits:

Each biscuit

Jaffa Cakes	*50 kcal*
Chocolate digestives	*100 kcal*
McVities Boasters	*88 kcal*

Fox's Millionaires	77 kcal
M & S Chocolate Vienenese Swirl	88 kcal
Jacobs shortbread finger	104 kcal
Kelloggs marshmallow square	132 kcal
Hob Nob bar	139 kcal
Penguin	136 kcal
Jacobs Club bar	133 kcal
Jordans Crunch bar	155 kcal
Cadbury chocolate fingers	29 kcal

HOME-MADE SHORTBREAD

Makes 8 pieces (226 kcal per piece)

Ingredients:

60g castor sugar	240 kcal
60g rice flour	230 kcal
1125g plain flour	425 kcal
125g butter	920 kcal
Total	**1815 Kcal**

Method:

Sift the dry ingredients into a bowl. Cut the butter into small cubes and rub in the sugar and flour until the mixture is evenly crumbly.

Press the crumbs together to form a ball and place on an oiled baking sheet. Flatten the ball to form a 20cm (8 inch) circle. Prick with a fork. Bake in an oven preheated to 180° for about 20 minutes until the shortbread is golden brown. Remove from the oven and cut into nine pieces whilst still hot. When they have cooled a little, they can be transferred to a wire rack to cool.

HAZELNUT BISCUITS

Makes 12 biscuits (218 kcal each)

Ingredients:

170g plain flour	580 kcal
85g castor sugar	340 kcal
1120g ground hazelnuts	780 kcal
125g butter	920 kcal
Total	**2620 kcal**

Method:

Beat the butter and sugar together until creamy. Add the flour and nuts and mix to a ball. Put the dough in the fridge for 30 minutes before rolling one to ¼" thick and cutting into 2½" circles with a cutter.

Place on an oiled backing sheet and cook in an oven preheated to 180° for 8–10 minutes. Remove from the oven and allow to cool a little before lifting them from the baking sheet.

Peanuts are an excellent food to snack on. They contain 250 kcal in 40g but beware, they are easily dropped down cushions and into pockets. Crisps are another good low-volume, high calorie-food.

Golden Wonder cheese & onion (34.5g)	*181 kcal per pack*
McCoys Thick & Crunchy (50g)	*255 kcal per pack*
Walkers (34.5g)	*186 kcal per pack*
Doritos Original (40g)	*210 kcal per pack*

M & S Prawn Crackers (50g)	269 kcal per pack
M & S Cheese Tasters (50g)	267 kcal per pack
McVities Mini Cheddars (35g)	187 kcal per pack
Kettle High Salted (50g)	248 kcal per pack
Pringles (35g) (5.5 kcal per Pringle)	193 kcal per pack

ICE CREAM

Ice cream and ice cream bars make good snacks. Here are some with the highest-calorie value.

Ben & Jerry's Chunky Munkey	240 kcal per 100g
Ben & Jerry's Bulker Almond Toffee Crunch	240 kcal per 100g
Häagen Daz Belgian Chocolate	270 kcal per 100g
Häagen Daz Macadonian Nut Brittle	240 kcal per 100g
Häagen Daz Praline & Cream	240 kcal per 100g

ICE CREAM BARS

Snickers	230 kcal each bar
Mars	210 kcal each bar
Twix	231 kcal each bar
Lion Bar	265 kcal each bar
Feast Bar	230 kcal each bar
Magnum Classic	295 kcal each bar
Magnum Almond	330 kcal each bar

Cakes make an easy snack and can be very high in calories. Here are some individual cakes which are high in calories:

M & S Fudge Brownie	236 kcal each cake
M & S Vanilla Slice	336 kcal each cake
M & S Egg Custard Tart	243 kcal each cake
Mr Kipling Luxury Mince Pies	244 kcal each cake
Mr Kipling Bramley Apple Pie	228 kcal each cake
Cadbury's Chocolate Flake Cake	242 kcal each cake

Large cakes that can be cut into portions:

M & S Chocolate Fudge Cake, 65g piece	260 kcal
M & S Country Cake, 65g piece	280 kcal
M & S Lemon Drizzle Cake, 65g piece	230 kcal

Cakes which you bake yourself are much higher in calories. Here are three which are particularly high. They can be cut into pieces and frozen if necessary.

AMERICAN BROWNIES

Makes 9 brownies (450 kcal each)

Ingredients:

250g chocolate	1,300 kcal
125g butter	920 kcal
2 eggs	160 kcal
140g sugar	560 kcal
35g plain flour	120 kcal
150g chopped walnuts	1,030 kcal
1tsp vanilla extract	

Method:

Gently melt the chocolate and butter together in a saucepan. Beat the eggs with the sugar until pale and frothy. Add the melted chocolate and butter to the egg mixture and stir in the sifted flour and the nuts. Add the vanilla.

Pour into an oiled 20cm-square baking tin and cook in an oven preheated to 190° for 25–30 minutes. The brownies are soft when you take them out of the oven and become firmer when they cool. Cut into nine pieces.

CARAMEL CRUNCH BISCUITS

(260 kcal each)

Ingredients:

1st layer:

100g butter	735 kcal
25g castor sugar	100 kcal
25g drinking chocolate powder	50 kcal
1 tsp vanilla essence	
175g digestive crumbled biscuits	460 kcal
50g chopped walnuts	340 kcal

2nd layer:

400g tin condensed milk	1,360 kcal
25g butter	180 kcal
3tbs golden syrup	120 kcal
100g milk chocolate	540 kcal
1tsp vanilla essence	

Method:

Brush a 7 x 11 inch swiss roll tin with the melted fat. To make the first layer, melt the butter, sugar, chocolate powder and vanilla essence in a saucepan over a low heat. Stir well.

Stir the crushed biscuits and chopped nuts into the melted mixture until all the fat has been absorbed. Press the mixture into the bottom of the swiss roll tin.

Tip all the second layer ingredients into a small heavy-based saucepan and heat gently until the mixture begins to bubble. Stir vigorously and continuously while the mixture boils for three minutes. A brown skin will form on the sides of the pan and this should be stirred in vigorously. Avoid letting the mixture burn.

Pour the caramel mixture over the biscuit base and spread evenly with a palette knife.

Place the chocolate in a small heatproof bowl and set the bowl over a pan of hot water. Stir until melted. Pour the chocolate over the caramel. Spread evenly and mark a pattern with the blunt side of the knife. Chill until set (about 2 hours).

Mark the chocolate into 15 equal squares. Cut in the tin using a sharp knife and life each square out with a palette knife.

N.B. Reproduced with the kind permission of Octopus Publishing Limited, *Chocolate Cooking* by Cathy Gill.

FRUIT CAKE

Makes 12 slices (420 kcal each)

Ingredients:

190g butter	1350 kcal
190g castor sugar	760 kcal
280g mixed dried fruit	790 kcal
380g self raising flour	1290 kcal
80g shredded almonds	550 kcal
3tbs milk	30 kcal
3 eggs	270 kcal

Method:

Place the sugar and flour into a bowl and add the butter cut into small cubes. Rub in the butter until the mixture resembles fine breadcrumbs. Add the milk and eggs and beat for 2–3 minutes. Add the dried fruit and almonds and stir well.

Place the mixture into a 20cm (8 inch) round cake tin lined with greaseproof paper.

Cook in an oven preheated to 180° for about ¼ hour. The cake is cooked when a skewer put into the centre remains clean when taken out. Leave the cake in the tin to cool a little before placing on a wire rack. The cake cuts into 12 slices.

LUNCH

Sandwiches make a quick and easy lunch. Two medium slices of bread with a normal covering of butter add up to 200 calories. In order to make a 500k-calorie sandwich you need to find fillings which add up to 300 calories.

Examples of 300-calorie fillings:

1.	1½tbs Mayonnaise	150 kcal
	100g chicken braest	150 kcal
2.	1½tbs Mayonnaise	150 kcal
	100g tinned tuna	150 kcal
3.	56g M&S coleslaw	100 kcal
	50g Cheddar cheese	200 kcal
4.	70g Philadelphia cream cheese	100 kcal
	1 large hard-boiled egg	100 kcal
5.	40g peanut butter	300 kcal
6.	55g Nutella	300 kcal

Ready-made sandwiches:

M & S Prawn & Mayonnaise	423 kcal
M & S Egg & Bacon	455 kcal
M & S Chicken & Sweetcorn	428 kcal
M & S Cheese & Celery	443 kcal
Waitrose Egg Mayonnaise	422 kcal
Waitrose Cheese Ploughmans	497 kcal
Waitrose Bacon, Lettuce & Tomato	448 kcal

You can make your own 500-calorie ploughmans lunch:

70g piece of French baguette	180 kcal
10g butter	72 kcal
30g pickle	40 kcal
50g hard cheese	208 kcal

You can make a sausage hotdog:

80g piece French baguette	*200 kcal*
1 pork sausage	*160 kcal*
60g fried onions	*110 kcal*
2tbs ketchup	*30 kcal*

Baked potatoes:

Baked potatoes make good lunchtime snacks. A medium potato provides about 200 calories so you need to put 300 calories of filling into it.

You could use any of the first four suggestions for sandwich fillings, i.e. grated cheese, cream cheese, chicken or tuna mayonnaise.

Pasta is a great favourite with children and is quick and easy to prepare.

75g pasta	*240 kcal*
15g butter	*120 kcal*
35g grated cheese	*140 kcal*

Cheese omelette is another quick lunch.

2 eggs	*180 kcal*
15g butter	*120 kcal*
50g grated cheese	*200 kcal*

Fry two whipped eggs in butter and add grated cheese.

Baked beans and cheese on toast is also high in calories.

2 medium slices of buttered toast	*200 kcal*
50g grated cheese	*200 kcal*
150g baked beans	*100 kcal*

Pitta bread is 155 kcal a piece. Taramasalata is 345 kcal. Together they make a 500-calorie lunch.

Some soups are very high in calories – here are some examples:

300ml Waitrose Chicken, Coconut with Lemon Grass	*300 kcal*
300ml M & S Potato and Leek soup	*300 kcal*
300ml New Covent Garden Spicy Corn Chowder	*350 kcal*

If you find a soup that is not quite high enough in calories, you can add double cream to it (1tbs 60 kcal)

Serve soups with 80g French bread or a buttered roll to make up the extra 200 calories.

Pizzas are very popular with children. Here are some high calorie pizzas:

½ Waitrose Bistro Salami and Pepperoni Pizza	*491 kcal*
M & S Store Baked Tomato and Cheese Pizza (312g)	*548 kcal*
½ Sainsbury Fresh Deep Pan 5 Cheese Feast (370g)	*514 kcal*
½ San Marco Margherita Pizza	*580 kcal*
½ Tesco Chicken and Bacon Pizza (448g)	*535 kcal*

If you find a pizza that is not quite high enough in calories, you can add grated cheese (15g adds 60 kcal).

Quiche served with or without baked beans makes a good lunch. M & S make individual quiches; their cheese and onion quiche (170g) is 502 kcal. Tesco make a 160g cornish pasty which is equally high in calories.

Surprisingly, it is possible to make high calorie salads. Here are some ideas:

FRENCH DRESSING

Ingredients:

1 tbs wine vinegar

3 tbs olive oil

½tsp sugar

½tsp french mustard

Salt & pepper

Method:

Mix ingredients in a screw top container and shake well. Shake again before using as it separates out quite easily.

Note: 1tbs of this dressing = 100 kcal

YOGHURT DRESSING

Ingredients:

2 tbs Greek yoghurt

1 tbs olive oil

½tsp French mustard

½tsp sugar

1tsb lemon juice

Salt & pepper

Method:

Mix ingredients in a screw top container and shake well.

Note: 1tbs of this dressing = 70 kcal

500-CALORIE CHEESE SALAD

Ingredients:

200g new potatoes	200 kcal
1 spring onion	nil kcal
2 tbs mayonnaise	200 kcal
25g grated Cheddar or hard cheese	100 kcal
Lettuce, cucumber, celery, peppers, etc	nil kcal

Method:

Slice the new potatoes and add chopped onion and mayonnaise. Serve with grated cheese and lettuce, cucumbers, peppers, etc.

500-CALORIE SALMON SALAD

Ingredients:

100g piece baked salmon	150 kcal
40g rice	150 kcal
60g canned sweetcorn	70 kcal
30g red pepper	nil kcal
15g raisins	30 kcal
1tbs French dressing	100 kcal
Lettuce, cucumber, celery, pepper, etc	nil kcal

Method:

Boil and cool the rice. Add the chopped red pepper, raisins and sweetcorn and stir in the French dressing. Serve with the salmon and lettuce, cucumber, etc.

500-CALORIE EGG SALAD

Ingredients:

2 hard boiled eggs	180 kcal
100g canned sweetcorn	100 kcal
1 tbs mayonnaise	150 kcal
2tbs Greek yoghurt	70 kcal
Lettuce, cucumber, celery, peppers, etc	nil kcal

Method:

Slice the eggs and add the corn, mayonnaise and yoghurt. Serve with lettuce, cucumber, tomatoes, etc.

500-CALORIE WALDORF SALAD

Ingredients:

2 sticks of celery	
large green apple	60 kcal
80g canned sweetcorn	100 kcal
10g chopped walnuts	70 kcal
2tbs mayonnaise	200 kcal
2tbs Greek yoghurt	70 kcal

Method:

Cut the celery and apple into small pieces. Add the sweetcorn and nuts. Mix in the yoghurt and mayonnaise. Serve with lettuce, tomato, cucumber, etc. The calorie content of these is negligible.

500-CALORIE CHICKEN SALAD

Ingredients:

1 roast chicken breast (approx. 100g)	155 kcal
50g M & S luxury coleslaw	150 kcal
½ medium avocado	95 kcal
1 small grated carrot	
1tbs French dressing	100 kcal
Lettuce, cucumber, celery, peppers, etc	nil kcal

Method:

Mix the grated carrot with the French dressing and serve with the chicken, avocado and coleslaw.

YOGHURTS

Greek yoghurts or wholemilk yoghurts provide the highest amount of calories. By using one of these which may have 200 calories a pot you could cut down the main snack by 50 calories. If you are using ordinary yoghurt, make sure that you are not buying those that are artificially sweetened. Most M & S fruit yoghurts have around 150 calories per pot.

If lunch is a real struggle or if you are in a rush, here is a recipe for a 700 kcalorie milkshake which fits a 250ml glass and can be drunk quickly.

100g Häagen Daz Vanilla or Toffee Crème Ice Cream	220 kcal
15g Nutella spread	80 kcal
30g smooth or crunchy peanut butter	180 kcal

2tbs / 30ml double cream	120 kcal
150ml full cream milk	100 kcal
	700 kcal

Put all the ingredients into a liquidiser and mix on full speed for 1 minutes. It tastes delicious and contains a lot of calories in a very small volume. It can replace the entire lunch.

MID AFTERNOON SNACK

One of the snacks, either morning or afternoon, should be a chocolate bar. All children love chocolate but I expect your anorexic child will try to convince you that she doesn't. If you insist that she eats a chocolate bar as part of her snacks every day she will realize that nothing terrible happens to her if she eats them. It is a great advantage if when she is travelling, or invariably misses a meal, she can eat a chocolate bar without flying into a panic. We always advise parents to make sure that their children take plenty of chocolate bars with them when they go on school trips as they invariably complain that they lost weight because there wasn't enough to eat. If they have a dozen Mars bars in their suitcase they have no excuse. Below is a list of the most popular chocolate bars. Don't be persuaded to cut bits off them to make them exactly the right number of calories. Explain that this is not abnormal behaviour. You can simply adjust one of the other meals to compensate for a chocolate bar, which has too many calories. If the bar is slightly under the calories needed, make the calories up with Ribena or fruit juice, don't leave yourself with a deficit to be made up later.

Anorexic children prefer Crunchies, Milkyways and KitKats

because they have a lower fat content than some of the other bars. Make sure that you buy lots of different bars and see that your child doesn't get into the habit of eating the same one every day.

CHOCOLATE BARS:
Cadbury Mars

Boost	*280 kcal*
Bounty	*270 kcal*
Caramel	*240 kcal*
47g Galaxy	*250 kcal*
Crunchie	*195 kcal*
65g Mars	*294 kcal*
Double Decker	*230 kcal*
52g twin Milky Way	*236 kcal*
Fruit & Nut standard bar	*240 kcal*
Topic	*234 kcal*
Picnic	*230 kcal*
62g Twin Twix	*307 kcal*
Starbar	*260 kcal*
Wispa	*210 kcal*

Nestlé

Aero Medium	*252 kcal*
Drifter twin	*270 kcal*
Kit Kat (4 finger)	*247 kcal*
Lion Bar	*247 kcal*
Toffee Crisp	*237 kcal*

EVENING MEAL

This is the biggest meal of the day and may need careful supervision. It may look like a lot of food but try to remember that this is just a temporary programme, to be followed because she is very thin. She will not always have to eat this much food and unless you are also very thin, you do not have to eat as much as she does.

It is important to try to serve high-calorie, low-volume food. The fat content is not important. It will not harm her if she eats a high-fat diet for a few weeks.

You can of course buy a calorie book and work out the exact number of calories in whatever meal you decide to cook. You do not have to prepare special food for her, you can simply bump up the calories of her portion by using extra butter, extra cream or extra cheese whenever you can.

Alternatively, you can serve her portion with chips, buttered rice or mashed potatoes. These are all high-calorie, low-volume foods which are ideal for children who have weight to gain.

100g medium cut chips deep fried	*320 kcal*
Roast potato medium piece	*50 kcal*
50g (uncooked) rice & 15g butter	*320 kcal*
200g (raw peeled weight) mashed potato	
with 15g butter	*400 kcal*
3oz sweetcorn & 15g butter	*200 kcal*
3oz fried onions	*150 kcal*
3ox fried aubergine	*250 kcal*

If you prefer not to cook, there are many very good and very high-calorie meals which you can buy ready made. Some of

them have sufficient calories on their own and some need
potatoes, rice or chips with them. Here are some suggestions:

Marks & Spencer

Macaroni Cheese 300g	495 kcal
Cannelloni 300g	480 kcal
Chicken Pasta Bake 300g	375 kcal
Sweet & Sour Chicken and Rice 400g	480 kcal
Bangers and Mash 369g	554 kcal
Haddock Mornay 400g	484 kcal
Roast Chicken Shortcrust Pie	476 kcal
Salmon En Croute	610 kcal
Cottage Pie 400g	500 kcal
Roast Lamb meal for one	765 kcal
Sausage and Onion filled Yorkshire Pud 320g	592 kcal

Waitrose

Tagliatelle Carbonara 300g	504 kcal
Chicken Kormu 340g	622 kcal
Chicken Biriyani 400g	732 kcal
Lamb Dopiaza 340g	510 kcal
Chicken Passanda 340g	629 kcal
Sweet & Sour Pork 300g	486 kcal
Salmon Rosti 300g	537 kcal
Moussaka 300g	506 kcal
Chicken Kiev	348 kcal
Fishermans Pie 300g	445 kcal
Shepherds Pie 400g	364 kcal

Tesco

Chicken Korma 300g	*690 kcal*
Toad in the Hole 170g	*617 kcal*
Chicken Biriyani & Rice 340g	*452 kcal*
Thai Red Chicken Curry 300g	*495 kcal*
Shepherds Pie 300g	*396 kcal*
Cottage Pie 300g	*558 kcal*
Chicken Tikka Masala 300g	*519 kcal*

Sainsbury

Chicken Dhansak with White Rice 450g	*465 kcal*
Duck in Plum Sauce with Noodles 450g	*504 kcal*
Sweet & Sour Chicken with Egg Fried Rice 450g	*657 kcal*
Creole Peanut Chicken with Cajun Rice 350g	*549 kcal*
Bengali Chicken 350g	*522 kcal*
Chicken Passanda 350g	*530 kcal*
Chicken Tikka Masala 350g	*572 kcal*
Corned Beef Hash 300g	*404 kcal*
Moussaka 500g	*810 kcal*

You can buy breaded dish, breaded chicken, sausages or any type of meat and serve with potatoes, rice or chips for a quick high-calorie meal.

If you have more time and you prefer to cook your own meals, here are some recipes which are high in calories.

The first two are quick sauce recipes which are laden with calories.

QUICK CHEESE SAUCE

Serves 4 (350 kcal per serving)

Ingredients:

275ml milk   275ml single cream

335g butter   35g cornflour

150g grated cheese   Salt and pepper

Method:

Boil the milk, cream and butter in a saucepan. Mix the corn flour with a little water until just liquid and add it to the boiling milk while you stir continuously. Boil for ½ minutes, remove from the heat and add the grated cheese. Season.

TOMATO SAUCE

Serves 4 (250 kcals per serving)

Ingredients:

1 medium tin tomatoes   1 medium sliced onion

1 clove garlic   125g butter

2tbs tomato purée   125ml stock made with a cube

Herbs, salt & pepper

Method:

Fry the onion and garlic in the butter until soft. Add tinned tomatoes, tomato purée and stock and liquidise. Add herbs and seasoning.

Both these sauces can be used to pour over pasta. You can add fish or meat to them and serve them with rice. You can add fish or meat and top with mashed potato and grated cheese to make a very high calorie pie.

In the plan we have suggested that you serve your child a 500-calorie main course and a 500-calorie dessert in order to give her 1,000 calories for her main meal. Most of the recipes included in this book are far higher than the 500 calories we suggest. You can either give your daughter much smaller portions, or alternate between a high-calorie main course with a light dessert such as ice cream or a high-calorie dessert with a very light main course such as a salad. The important point is that the main course and dessert add up to 1,000 kcal.

RICH ONION QUICHE

Serves 6 (517 kcal each serving)
Ingredients:

Pastry:
160g plain flour
110g butter
1 egg yolk

Filling:
30g butter
2 large onions
100g Cheddar cheese
150ml double cream
3 eggs
Salt and pepper

Method:
Mix the flour and butter for the pastry in a food processor. Add the egg yolk, with 2–3 tsp of water if necessary, to form a ball which can be rolled out. Roll the pastry on a floured board and line a 20cm (8 inch) flan case. Line the pastry with greaseproof paper and fill with rice or beans. Bake in a oven preheated to

220° C for 15 - 20 minutes. Remove from the oven, take out the greaseproof paper and beans and allow to cool. Fry the chopped onions in the butter until soft. Remove from the pan and allow to cool. Place the 3 eggs and cream in a bowl and beat well for one minute. Season. Spread the onions over the bottom of the pastry case and put in the egg mixture. Bake in an oven preheated to 160° C for 35–40 minutes until the flan is set.

CHICKEN PASTA BAKE

Serves 4 (684 kcal each serving)

Ingredients:

250g fresh pasta	*2 skinned chicken breasts*
1 tin of tomatoes	*100g sweetcorn*
50g grated Cheddar cheese	*1 'quick cheese sauce recipe'*
	(page 159)

Method:

Bake the chicken breasts in the oven at 200° C for approximately 15 minutes until cooked. Boil the pasta until cooked. Heat the drained chopped tomatoes and sweetcorn in a saucepan or in the microwave. Put the hot drained pasta together with the tomato, sweetcorn and chopped hot chicken breasts into an ovenproof dish. Pour over the hot cheese sauce. Sprinkle with the grated cheese and place under the grill for 2–3 minutes to brown.

SWEET & SOUR CHICKEN

Serves 4 (400 kcal each serving)

Ingredients:

Sauce:

1tbs sugar	*4 chicken breasts*
1tbs soy sauce	*1 beaten egg*
1tsp grated root ginger	*Cornflour*
150ml water	*8tbs oil*
2tbs vinegar	
2tbs fresh orange juice	
1tbs cornflour	
1tbs tomato puree	

Method:

Mix the cornflour to a paste with some of the water. Mix the paste with all the other ingredients for the sauce in a saucepan and bring to the boil whilst stirring constantly. Cut the chicken breasts into cubes, dip in the beaten egg and roll in the cornflour. Fry in the oil until golden brown. When the chicken is cooked, remove the pieces of chicken from the frying pan, pour over the sauce and serve.

CHICKEN RISOTTO

Serves 4 (544 kcal each serving)

Ingredients:

200g risotto rice	*1 clove of garlic*
100g butter	*1 litre of chicken stock*
2 medium onions	*2 skinned chicken breasts*
100g sweetcorn	*50g grated Parmesan cheese*

Method:

Melt the butter and fry the onions and garlic until soft. Add the chopped chicken and stir until cooked. Add the rice and stir for a couple of minutes. Add the stock while stirring constantly. Cover and simmer on a very low heat, stirring frequently to prevent sticking. When all the liquid has been absorbed and the rice is cooked, add the sweetcorn and Parmesan cheese. Stir for a few more moments being careful to see that the rice does not stick to the bottom of the saucepan.

CHICKEN EN CROUTE

Serves 4 (830 kcal each serving)

Ingredients:

2 *medium chopped onions*	*4tbs oil*
1 *chopped clove garlic*	*30g butter*
4 *chopped rashers of smoked bacon*	*400g puff pastry*
4 *skinned chicken breasts*	*1 beaten egg*

Method:

Heat the oil in a frying pan and cook the chicken breasts until sealed. Remove and leave to cool. Add butter to the remaining oil and fry the chopped onions and garlic until soft. Add bacon and continue to cook for 3–4 minutes. Remove from pan and cool.

Cut the pastry into four and roll out into four rectangles large enough to cover the chicken. Place the breasts on one half of the pastry and add a quarter of the onion/bacon mix to the top of each. Brush the egg onto the edge of the pastry fold over and seal. Brush the top with the remaining egg and make two cuts in the pastry to release any steam. Cook in an oven preheated to 200°C for approximately 30 minutes.

SATÉ CHICKEN

Serves 4 (546 kcal each serving)

Ingredients:

1 medium onion

1 clove garlic

Juice of ½ lemon

1tsb soya sauce

4 skinned chicken breasts

250g roasted peanuts

1tsp brown sugar

280ml coconut milk

1 level tsp chilli powder

Method:

Place onion, garlic clove, sugar, peanuts and chilli powder in a liquidiser and turn for 2–3 minutes. Place the ingredients in a frying pan and dry fry for a few moments. Add the lemon juice and stir well. Add the coconut milk and bring to the boil. Simmer until thick, then pour the sauce over the grilled chicken breasts.

SALMON FISH PIE

Serves 4 (1,068 kcal each serving)

Ingredients:

600g skinless salmon fillet

100ml double cream

85g butter

300ml full cream milk

500g grated Cheddar cheese

For mashed potato:

100ml double cream

750g potato

85g butter

Method:

Poach the salmon in the 300ml of milk plus 100ml of double cream for 8 minutes until cooked. Remove with a slotted spoon and place in an ovenproof dish. Flake the salmon so as to cover the bottom of the dish. Add 85g butter to the milk and cream mixture and heat. Mix the cornflour with a little water until just liquid. Add to the boiling milk mixture and stir well until thickened. Add salt and pepper and pour over the salmon in the dish. Boil the potatoes until soft. Drain the water and mash well with the remaining butter and the remaining 100ml of double cream. Spread the potato mixture over the salmon and sauce in the dish. Sprinkle with the grated cheese. Cook in an oven preheated to 200°C for 30 minutes.

SALMON FISH CAKES

Serves 4 (448 kcal each serving)

Ingredients:

350g salmon	*300g peeled potatoes*
2 level tbs double cream	*1 medium egg beaten*
1 large grated onion	*500g sweetcorn*
1tsp lemon juice	*80g fine white bread crumbs*
Salt and pepper	*4tbs oil to fry*

Method:

Loosely wrap the salmon in foil and place in an oven preheated to 200°C for approximately 15 minutes until cooked. Boil the potatoes and mash. Do not add butter or milk. Place the mashed potatoes in a bowl and mix in the flaked salmon, double cream, beaten egg, grated onion and lemon juice. Mix well. Divide the mixture into 8 round fishcakes. Press the fishcakes one by one into the breadcrumbs until completely covered. Heat the oil in a large frying pan and fry the fishcakes for approximately 3 minutes each side until browned.

RASPBERRY TRIFLE

Serves 6 (556 kcal each serving)

Ingredients:

1 jam swiss roll

1 packet of M & S thick and creamy custard

½ml of double cream

225g fresh or frozen raspberries

1 raspberry jelly

1 Cadbury's flake bar

Method:

Cut the swiss roll into six and place in the bottom of a glass bowl. Pour on the cooled jelly mixture and put in the fridge to set. Whip the double cream until just stiff and fold into the custard. Spoon on top of the jelly. Once set and sprinkle with the crumbled flake.

PECAN PIE

Serves 6 (755 kcal each serving)

Ingredients:

Pastry:

175g plain flour

125g butter

1 egg yolk

2–3 tsp water

Filling:

3 medium eggs

200g golden syrup

100g soft brown sugar

40g butter

180g chopped pecan nuts

50g halved pecan nuts

Method:

Rub the butter into the plain flour. Mix in the egg yolk and water to form a ball. Put in the fridge and chill for 30 minutes. Use it once cool to line a 20cm (8 inch) flan case. Put the chopped pecan nuts into the pastry case. Whisk the eggs until light, add the syrup, melted butter and sugar. Whisk together again and pour into the pastry case. Place the pecan halves on top and place in an oven preheated to 190°C for 25–30 minutes.

APPLE CRUMBLE

Serves 4 (428 kcal each serving)

Ingredients:

75g flour	*50g ground hazelnuts*
75g brown sugar	*50g butter*
600g eating apples	*50g sugar*

Method:

Peel, core and slice the apples into an ovenproof dish and sprinkle with 50g of sugar. Rub the flour and 50g butter together until it resembles fine breadcrumbs. Add brown sugar and ground nuts and mix well. Spoon the crumble mixture over the apples and cook in an oven preheated to 190°C for 25–30 minutes.

BAKEWELL TART

Serves 4 (489 kcal each serving)

Ingredients: **Filling:**

175g plain flour	*3tbs raspberry jam*
125g butter	*50g butter*
1 egg yolk	*50g castor sugar*
2–3 tsp water	*1 beaten egg*
	50g ground almonds
	50g cake crumbs
	Grated rind of ½ lemon

Method:

Rub flour and butter together and add egg yolk and water to form a ball. Chill in the fridge for half and hour before rolling into a 20cm (8 inch) flan dish. Prick the base with a fork. Cover in jam. Cream the butter and castor sugar and gradually beat in the egg. Fold in the ground almonds, cake crumbs and grated rind. Spoon over the jam and cook in an oven preheated to 180° for 25–30 minutes.

APPLE SPONGE

Serves 4 (772 kcal each serving)

Ingredients:

4 eating apples	*1 tin of condensed milk*
85g butter	*85g castor sugar*
1 large egg	*150g self raising flour*

Method:

Peel, core and slice the apples. Poach in a pan with 2 tbs of water until just soft . Place the unopened tin of condensed milk in half a pan of water and boil gently with the lid on for 3 hours. Take great care not to allow the saucepan to boil dry.

Beat the sugar and butter together until very light. Whisk in the beaten egg a little at a time. Fold in the flour and add two or three tablespoons of milk until the mixture drops from the spoon. Place the apple pieces in a small ovenproof dish, cover with the boiled condensed milk and spread the sponge mixture over the top. Bake in an oven preheated to 180° for about 40 minutes.

CHEESECAKE

Serves 6 (520 kcal each serving)

Ingredients:

75g butter   125g digestive biscuits

125g mascapone   100g cream cheese

125ml double cream   2 eggs

50g castor sugar   grated rind and juice of
                              1 lemon

Method:

Put the melted butter and biscuits into a food processor and spin until crushed. Press the buttered crumbs into the base of a 20cm (8 inch) flan case. Whisk all the remaining ingredients together and pour into the tin. Bake in the middle of an oven preheated to 150° for about 1½ hours or until just set.

TIRAMISU

Serves 4 (624 kcal each serving)

Ingredients:

160g plain sponge cake   140ml maple syrup

40ml water   150g mascapone

150ml double cream   1 chocolate flake

4 mini meringues   60g icing sugar

Method:

Cut the cake into pieces and lay in the bottom of a glass bowl. Mix the maple syrup and water together and pour over the cake to soak it. Whisk the double cream until stiff and fold in the muscapone and icing sugar. Spoon over the sponge cake.

Sprinkle with crumbled mini meringues and the chocolate flake. Refrigerate for 2 hours before serving.

BREAD AND BUTTER PUDDING

Serves 4 (705 kcal each serving)

Ingredients:

3 hot cross buns	*35g butter*
25g sultanas	*300ml milk*
30ml double cream	*2 eggs*
50g sugar	*1tsp vanilla extract*

Method:

Cut the hot cross buns in half and butter with 35g butter. Place in the bottom of an ovenproof dish and sprinkle with the sultanas. Mix the milk, cream, eggs, sugar and vanilla together and whisk for a minute. Pour the mixture over the hot cross buns. Place the ovenproof dish inside a baking dish and pour water in until it comes half way up the side of the dish. Bake in an oven preheated to 180°C for 35–40 minutes until just browned.

CHOCOLATE MOUSSE

Serves 6 (458 kcal each serving)

Ingredients:

180g dark chocolate

280ml double cream

50g butter

4 eggs

Method:

Separate the eggs. Melt the chocolate and butter very gently in a pan and beat the egg yolks in one at a time with an electric whisk. Beat the egg whites until just stiff and fold into the chocolate mixture. Spoon into a glass bowl and chill for 2 hours before serving.

SYRUP SPONGE

Serves 4 (631 kcal each serving)

Ingredients:

200g self raising flour	*2 eggs*
100g castor sugar	*Milk*
100g butter	*6 tbs golden syrup*

Method:

Rub the butter into the flour and add the sugar. Whisk the eggs and mix into the flour mixture until smooth. Add a little milk if necessary to make the mixture just drop from the spoon. Grease a basin which can be boiled and put 3tbs of golden syrup into the bottom. Add half the sponge mixture. Spoon the remaining 3tbs of golden syrup over the sponge mixture and cover with the remaining mix. Cover well with a lid or foiled secured with string. Place in a steamer for about 1½ hours.

Average weight charts

Research carried out at Great Ormond Street Hospital for sick children has shown that the majority of girls menstruate and function normally if they are 5% below the average weight for their age and height.

As we know that anorexic children want to be as thin as possible, we set their target weight at 95% of an average weight. Of course your daughter could be 10 – 15% above this weight and still be within normal limits.

If your child has stabilised for 6 months at her 95% weight and has not regained her periods, she may need to have her weight raised to 100%. It is possible to ask your doctor to arrange an ovarian scan if her periods do not return.

We must stress that the 95% weight given in these charts are the very minimum that your child should be.

It is safe for boys to be at the 95% level although because of their much lower body fat they look extremely thin at these weights. The 100% weight is preferable for boys even though it is not medically necessary.

If your daughter is 13 years old and her height is 150cm you will see that her minimum weight should be 40.8kg. When consulting the chart, always round your daughter's age up and not down. Remember that as she grows and gets older, you will need to recalculate her target weight.

If you want to calculate her present percentage you can do so as follows:

First you must calculate her 100% weight. To do this, you must take her 95% weight from the chart, divide it by 95 and multiply it by 100.

If your child has a 95% weight of 40.8kg:

$$\frac{40.8\text{kg}}{95} \times 100 = 43\text{kg}.$$

Her 100% weight would be 43kg. If she currently weighs only 32.25kg you can calculate her current percentage like this:

$$\frac{\text{Present weight}}{100\% \text{ weight}} \times 100 \qquad \frac{32.25 \text{ kg}}{43 \text{ kg}} \times 100 = 75\%$$

This shows a child who is only 75% of a normal weight and unless she is gaining a steady amount of weight each week should be hospitalised. As she gains weight you can recalculate her current percentage and allow her a little more exercise as she approaches target weight.

	148 cm	149 cm	150 cm	151 cm	152 cm	153 cm	154 cm	155 cm	156 cm	157 cm	158 cm	159 cm	160 cm	161 cm	162 cm	163 cm	164 cm	165 cm	166 cm	167 cm	168 cm
10 yrs 0 mths	34.0	34.5	35.0	35.0	35.5	36.0	36.5	37.5	38.0	38.5	39.0	39.5	40.0	40.5	41.0	41.5	42.0	42.5	43.0	43.5	44.0
10 yrs 0 mths	34.5	34.5	35.0	35.5	36.0	36.5	37.5	38.0	38.5	39.0	39.5	40.0	40.5	41.0	41.5	42.0	42.5	43.0	43.5	44.0	44.5
10 yrs 3 mths	34.5	35.0	35.0	36.0	36.5	37.0	37.5	38.0	38.5	39.0	39.5	40.0	40.5	41.0	41.5	42.0	42.5	43.0	43.5	44.0	44.0
10 yrs 6 mths	34.5	35.5	36.0	36.5	37.0	37.5	38.0	38.5	39.0	39.5	40.0	40.5	41.0	41.5	42.0	42.5	43.0	43.5	44.0	44.5	45.0
10 yrs 6 mths	35.0	35.5	36.0	36.5	37.0	37.5	38.0	38.5	39.0	39.5	40.0	40.5	41.0	41.5	42.0	42.5	43.0	43.5	44.0	44.5	45.0
10 yrs 9 mths	35.0	36.0	36.5	37.0	37.5	38.0	38.5	39.0	39.5	40.0	40.5	41.0	41.5	42.0	42.5	43.0	43.5	44.0	44.5	45.0	45.5
11 yrs 0 mths	35.0	36.0	36.5	37.0	37.5	38.5	39.0	39.5	40.0	40.5	41.0	41.5	42.0	42.5	43.0	43.5	44.0	44.5	45.0	45.5	46.0
11 yrs 0 mths	35.0	36.5	37.0	37.5	38.0	38.5	39.0	39.5	40.0	40.5	41.0	41.5	42.5	43.0	43.5	44.0	44.5	45.0	45.5	46.0	46.5
11 yrs 3 mths	35.0	36.5	37.0	37.5	38.5	39.0	39.5	40.0	40.5	41.0	41.5	42.0	42.5	43.0	43.5	44.0	44.5	45.0	45.5	46.0	46.5
11 yrs 3 mths	35.5	37.0	37.5	38.0	38.5	39.0	39.5	40.0	40.5	41.0	41.5	42.0	42.5	43.0	43.5	44.0	44.5	45.5	46.0	46.5	47.0
11 yrs 6 mths	35.5	37.0	37.5	38.0	38.5	39.0	39.5	40.5	41.0	41.5	42.0	42.5	43.0	43.5	44.0	44.5	45.0	45.5	46.5	47.0	47.5
11 yrs 9 mths	36.0	37.0	38.0	38.5	39.0	39.5	40.0	40.5	41.0	41.5	42.0	42.5	43.0	43.5	44.0	44.5	45.5	46.0	46.5	47.0	48.0
12 yrs 0 mths	36.0	37.5	38.5	39.0	39.5	40.0	40.5	41.0	41.5	42.0	42.5	43.0	43.5	44.0	45.0	45.5	46.0	46.5	47.0	48.0	48.5
12 yrs 3 mths	36.5	37.5	38.5	39.0	39.5	40.0	40.5	41.0	41.5	42.0	42.5	43.0	44.0	44.5	45.0	45.5	46.0	46.5	47.5	48.0	48.5
12 yrs 3 mths	37.0	38.0	39.0	39.5	40.0	40.5	41.0	41.5	42.0	42.5	43.0	43.5	44.0	44.5	45.0	45.5	46.5	47.0	47.5	48.0	49.0
12 yrs 6 mths	37.0	38.0	39.0	39.5	40.0	40.5	41.0	41.5	42.0	42.5	43.0	44.0	44.5	45.0	45.5	46.0	46.5	47.0	48.0	48.5	49.5
12 yrs 9 mths	37.5	38.5	39.5	40.0	40.5	41.0	41.5	42.0	42.5	43.0	43.5	44.0	44.5	45.0	46.0	46.5	47.0	47.5	48.0	49.0	50.0
13 yrs 0 mths	37.5	39.0	39.5	40.0	40.5	41.5	42.0	42.5	43.0	43.5	44.0	44.5	45.0	46.0	46.5	47.0	47.5	48.0	48.5	49.5	50.5
13 yrs 3 mths	38.0	39.0	40.0	40.5	41.0	41.5	42.0	42.5	43.0	43.5	44.0	44.5	45.5	46.0	46.5	47.0	47.5	48.5	49.0	50.0	51.0
13 yrs 3 mths	38.0	39.5	40.0	40.5	41.5	42.0	42.5	43.0	43.5	44.0	44.5	45.0	45.5	46.5	47.0	47.5	48.0	48.5	49.5	50.5	51.5
13 yrs 6 mths	38.0	39.5	40.5	41.0	41.5	42.0	42.5	43.5	44.0	44.5	45.0	45.5	46.0	46.5	47.0	48.0	48.5	49.0	50.0	50.5	52.0
13 yrs 9 mths	38.5	40.0	40.5	41.5	42.0	42.5	43.0	43.5	44.5	45.0	45.5	46.0	46.5	47.0	47.5	48.0	49.0	49.5	50.0	51.0	52.5
14 yrs 0 mths	39.0	40.0	41.0	41.5	42.0	43.0	43.5	44.0	44.5	45.0	46.0	46.5	47.0	47.5	48.0	48.5	49.5	50.0	50.5	51.5	52.5
14 yrs 3 mths	39.0	40.5	41.5	42.0	42.5	43.0	44.0	44.5	45.0	45.5	46.0	47.0	47.5	48.0	48.5	49.0	50.0	50.5	51.0	52.0	53.0
14 yrs 3 mths	39.5	40.5	41.0	42.0	42.5	43.5	44.0	44.5	45.0	46.0	46.5	47.0	47.5	48.0	49.0	49.5	50.0	51.0	51.5	52.5	53.0
14 yrs 6 mths	39.5	41.0	42.0	42.5	43.0	44.0	44.5	45.0	46.0	46.5	47.0	47.5	48.5	49.0	49.5	50.0	50.5	51.5	52.0	53.0	53.5
14 yrs 9 mths	40.0	41.0	42.0	43.0	43.5	44.0	45.0	45.5	46.0	46.5	47.5	48.0	48.5	49.0	50.0	50.5	51.0	52.0	52.5	53.5	54.0
15 yrs 0 mths	40.0	41.5	42.5	43.0	44.0	44.5	45.0	45.5	46.5	47.0	47.5	48.0	49.0	49.5	50.0	51.0	51.5	52.0	53.0	53.5	54.5
15 yrs 0 mths	40.5	41.5	42.5	43.0	44.0	44.5	45.0	46.0	46.5	47.5	48.0	48.5	49.5	50.0	50.5	51.5	52.0	52.5	53.0	54.0	55.0
15 yrs 3 mths	40.5	42.0	42.5	43.5	44.5	45.0	45.5	46.5	47.0	47.5	48.5	49.0	50.0	50.5	51.0	52.0	52.5	53.0	54.0	54.5	55.5
15 yrs 6 mths	41.0	42.0	43.0	44.0	44.5	45.5	46.0	46.5	47.5	48.0	48.5	49.5	50.0	51.0	51.5	52.0	53.0	53.5	54.5	55.0	56.0
15 yrs 6 mths	41.0	42.5	43.0	44.0	45.0	45.5	46.0	47.0	47.5	48.5	49.0	50.0	50.5	51.0	52.0	52.5	53.5	54.0	55.0	55.5	56.5
15 yrs 9 mths	41.0	42.5	43.5	44.5	45.0	46.0	46.5	47.5	48.0	49.0	49.5	50.5	51.0	52.0	52.5	53.0	54.0	55.0	55.5	56.5	
16 yrs 0 mths	41.5	42.5	43.5	44.0	45.0	45.5	46.5	47.0	48.0	48.5	49.5	50.0	51.0	51.5	52.5	53.0	54.0	54.5	55.5	56.0	
16 yrs 0 mths	42.0	42.5	43.5	44.5	45.0	46.0	46.5	47.5	48.0	49.0	49.5	50.5	51.0	52.0	52.5	53.5	54.0	55.0	55.5		
17 yrs 0 mths	43.0	43.5	44.0	45.0	45.5	46.5	47.0	47.5	48.5	49.0	50.0	50.5	51.5	52.0	53.0	53.5	54.5	55.0			
18 yrs 0 mths	43.0	43.5	44.0	45.0	45.5	46.0	47.0	48.0	48.5	49.5	50.0	51.0	52.0	52.5	53.5	54.0	54.5				
18 yrs 0 mths	44.0	44.5	45.0	45.5	46.0	47.0	47.5	48.0	48.5	49.0	50.0	50.5	51.0	52.0	53.0	53.5	54.5	55.0			

BOYS

	127 cm	128 cm	129 cm	130 cm	131 cm	132 cm	133 cm	134 cm	135 cm	136 cm	137 cm	138 cm	139 cm	140 cm	141 cm	142 cm	143 cm	144 cm	145 cm	146 cm	147 cm
10 yrs 0 mths	25.0	25.5	26.0	26.5	27.0	27.0	27.5	28.0	28.5	29.0	29.0	29.5	30.0	30.5	31.0	31.5	32.0	32.5	33.0	33.5	34.0
10 yrs 3 mths	25.0	25.5	26.0	26.5	27.0	27.5	27.5	28.0	28.5	29.0	29.5	30.0	30.0	30.5	31.0	31.5	32.0	32.5	33.0	33.5	34.0
10 yrs 6 mths	25.5	26.0	26.5	27.0	27.0	27.5	28.0	28.5	29.0	29.0	30.0	30.0	30.5	31.0	31.5	32.0	32.5	33.0	33.5	34.0	34.0
10 yrs 9 mths	25.5	26.0	26.5	27.0	27.5	27.5	28.0	28.5	29.0	29.5	30.0	30.5	31.0	31.0	31.5	32.0	32.5	33.0	33.5	34.0	34.5
11 yrs 0 mths	26.0	26.0	27.0	27.0	27.5	28.0	28.5	29.0	29.0	29.5	30.0	30.5	31.0	31.5	32.0	32.0	33.0	33.5	34.0	34.5	34.5
11 yrs 3 mths	26.0	26.5	27.0	27.5	28.0	28.0	28.5	29.0	29.5	30.0	30.0	30.5	31.0	31.5	32.0	32.5	33.0	33.5	34.0	34.5	35.0
11 yrs 6 mths	26.0	27.0	27.0	27.5	28.0	28.5	29.0	29.5	29.5	30.0	30.5	31.0	31.5	32.0	32.5	33.0	33.5	34.0	34.5	35.0	35.0
11 yrs 9 mths	26.0	27.0	27.5	28.0	28.0	28.5	29.0	29.5	30.0	30.5	31.0	31.5	32.0	32.0	32.5	33.0	33.5	34.0	34.5	35.0	35.0
12 yrs 0 mths	27.5	28.0	28.0	28.5	29.0	29.0	29.5	30.0	30.5	31.0	31.0	31.5	32.0	32.5	33.0	33.0	33.5	34.0	34.5	35.0	35.5
12 yrs 3 mths	27.0	27.5	28.0	28.5	29.0	29.5	30.0	30.0	30.5	31.0	31.5	32.0	32.0	32.5	33.0	33.5	34.0	34.5	35.0	35.0	35.5
12 yrs 6 mths	27.5	28.0	28.5	29.0	29.0	29.5	30.0	30.5	31.0	31.0	32.0	32.0	32.5	33.0	33.5	34.0	34.5	35.0	35.0	35.5	36.0
12 yrs 9 mths	27.5	28.0	28.5	29.0	29.5	30.0	30.0	30.5	31.0	31.5	32.0	32.5	33.0	33.0	33.5	34.0	34.5	35.0	35.5	36.0	36.0
13 yrs 0 mths	28.0	28.5	29.0	29.5	30.0	30.0	30.5	31.0	31.5	32.0	32.0	32.5	33.0	33.5	34.0	34.0	35.0	35.5	36.0	37.0	37.5
13 yrs 3 mths	28.0	28.5	29.0	29.5	30.0	30.5	31.0	31.0	31.5	32.0	32.5	33.0	33.0	33.5	34.0	34.5	35.0	35.5	36.0	37.5	38.0
13 yrs 6 mths	28.0	29.0	29.0	29.5	30.0	30.5	31.0	31.5	32.0	32.0	33.0	33.0	33.5	34.0	34.5	35.0	35.5	36.0	37.0	37.5	38.0
13 yrs 9 mths	28.0	29.0	29.5	30.0	30.0	30.5	31.0	31.5	32.0	32.5	33.0	33.5	34.0	34.0	34.5	35.0	35.5	36.0	37.5	38.0	38.5
14 yrs 0 mths	29.0	29.5	30.0	30.5	31.0	31.0	31.5	32.0	32.5	33.0	33.0	33.5	34.0	34.5	35.0	35.0	36.0	36.5	37.0	38.0	39.0
14 yrs 3 mths	29.5	30.0	30.5	31.0	31.5	31.5	32.0	32.5	33.0	33.5	34.0	34.0	34.5	35.0	35.5	36.0	36.5	37.0	37.5	38.5	39.5
14 yrs 6 mths	30.0	30.0	30.5	31.0	31.5	32.0	32.5	33.0	33.5	34.0	34.0	34.5	35.0	35.5	36.0	36.5	37.0	37.5	38.0	39.0	40.0
14 yrs 9 mths	30.0	30.0	31.0	31.5	32.0	32.5	32.5	33.0	33.5	34.0	34.5	35.0	35.5	36.0	36.5	37.0	37.5	38.0	38.5	39.5	40.0
15 yrs 0 mths	30.0	30.5	31.0	31.5	32.0	32.5	33.0	33.5	34.0	34.5	35.0	35.5	36.0	36.5	37.0	37.5	38.0	38.5	39.0	40.0	40.5
15 yrs 3 mths	30.5	31.0	31.5	32.0	32.5	33.0	33.5	34.0	34.5	35.0	35.5	36.0	36.5	37.0	37.5	38.0	38.5	39.0	39.5	40.0	40.5
15 yrs 6 mths	30.5	31.0	31.5	32.0	33.0	33.5	34.0	34.5	35.0	35.5	36.0	36.5	37.0	37.5	38.0	38.5	39.0	39.5	40.0	40.5	41.0
15 yrs 9 mths	31.0	31.5	32.0	32.5	33.0	33.5	34.0	34.5	35.0	35.5	36.0	36.5	37.0	37.5	38.0	38.5	39.0	39.5	40.0	40.5	41.5
16 yrs 0 mths	31.0	31.5	32.0	32.5	33.0	34.0	34.5	35.0	35.5	36.0	36.5	37.0	37.5	38.0	38.5	39.0	39.5	40.0	40.5	41.0	41.5
17 yrs 0 mths	31.5	32.0	32.5	33.0	33.5	34.0	34.5	35.0	35.5	36.0	36.5	37.0	37.5	38.5	39.0	39.5	40.0	40.5	41.0	42.0	42.5
18 yrs 0 mths	32.0	32.5	33.0	33.5	34.0	34.5	35.0	35.5	36.0	36.5	37.0	37.5	38.0	39.0	39.5	40.5	41.0	41.5	42.0	42.5	43.0

	127 cm	128 cm	129 cm	130 cm	131 cm	132 cm	133 cm	134 cm	135 cm	136 cm	137 cm	138 cm	139 cm	140 cm	141 cm	142 cm	143 cm	144 cm	145 cm	146 cm	147 cm
10 yrs 0 mths	26.0	26.0	26.5	27.0	27.5	28.0	28.5	29.0	29.5	30.0	30.5	31.0	31.5	32.0	32.5	33.0	33.5	34.0	34.5	35.0	35.5
10 yrs 3 mths	26.0	26.5	27.0	27.5	28.0	28.5	29.0	29.5	30.0	30.0	30.5	31.0	31.5	32.0	32.5	33.0	33.5	34.0	34.5	35.0	35.0
10 yrs 6 mths	26.5	26.5	27.0	27.5	28.0	28.5	29.0	29.5	29.5	30.0	30.5	31.0	31.5	32.0	32.5	33.0	33.5	34.0	34.5	35.0	35.5
10 yrs 9 mths	26.5	27.0	27.5	27.5	28.0	28.5	29.0	29.5	30.0	30.5	31.0	31.5	32.0	32.5	33.0	33.5	34.0	34.5	35.0	35.5	36.0
11 yrs 0 mths	26.5	27.0	27.5	28.0	28.5	29.0	29.5	30.0	30.5	30.5	31.0	31.5	32.0	32.5	33.0	33.5	34.0	34.5	35.0	35.5	36.0
11 yrs 3 mths	27.0	27.5	28.0	28.0	28.5	29.0	29.5	30.0	30.5	31.0	31.5	32.0	32.0	32.5	33.0	33.5	34.0	34.5	35.0	35.5	36.0
11 yrs 6 mths	27.0	27.5	28.0	28.5	29.0	29.5	30.0	30.5	31.0	31.0	31.5	32.0	32.5	33.0	33.5	34.0	34.5	35.0	35.5	36.0	36.5
11 yrs 9 mths	27.5	27.5	28.0	28.5	29.0	29.5	30.0	30.5	31.0	31.5	32.0	32.5	33.0	33.5	34.0	34.5	35.0	35.5	36.0	36.5	37.0
12 yrs 0 mths	27.5	28.0	28.5	29.0	29.5	30.0	30.5	31.0	31.5	32.0	32.5	33.0	33.5	34.0	34.5	35.0	35.5	36.0	36.5	37.0	37.5
12 yrs 3 mths	28.0	28.5	29.0	29.0	29.5	30.0	30.5	31.0	31.5	32.0	32.5	33.0	33.5	34.0	34.5	35.0	35.5	36.0	36.5	37.0	37.5
12 yrs 6 mths	28.0	28.5	29.0	29.5	30.0	30.5	31.0	31.5	32.0	32.5	33.0	33.5	34.0	34.5	35.0	35.5	36.0	36.5	37.0	37.5	38.0
12 yrs 9 mths	28.0	28.5	29.0	29.5	30.0	30.5	31.0	31.5	32.0	32.5	33.0	33.5	34.0	34.5	35.0	35.5	36.0	36.5	37.0	37.5	38.0
13 yrs 0 mths	28.5	29.0	29.5	30.0	30.5	31.0	31.5	32.0	32.5	33.0	33.5	34.0	34.5	35.0	35.5	36.0	36.5	37.0	37.5	38.0	38.5
13 yrs 3 mths	29.0	29.5	30.0	30.5	31.0	31.5	32.0	32.5	33.0	33.5	34.0	34.5	35.0	35.5	36.0	36.5	37.0	37.5	38.0	38.5	39.0
13 yrs 6 mths	29.5	30.0	30.5	31.0	31.5	32.0	32.5	33.0	33.5	34.0	34.5	35.0	35.5	36.0	36.5	37.0	37.5	38.0	38.5	39.0	39.5
13 yrs 9 mths	29.5	30.0	30.5	31.0	31.5	32.0	32.5	33.0	33.5	34.0	34.5	35.0	35.5	36.0	36.5	37.0	37.5	38.0	38.5	39.0	39.5
14 yrs 0 mths	30.0	30.5	31.0	31.5	32.0	32.5	33.0	33.5	34.0	34.5	35.0	35.5	36.0	36.5	37.0	37.5	38.0	38.5	39.0	39.5	40.0
14 yrs 3 mths	30.5	31.0	31.5	32.0	32.5	33.0	33.5	34.0	34.5	35.0	35.5	36.0	36.5	37.0	37.5	38.0	38.5	39.0	39.5	40.0	40.5
14 yrs 6 mths	31.0	31.5	32.0	32.5	33.0	33.5	34.0	34.5	35.0	35.5	36.0	36.5	37.0	37.5	38.0	38.5	39.0	39.5	40.0	40.5	41.0
14 yrs 9 mths	31.0	31.5	32.0	32.5	33.0	33.5	34.0	34.5	35.0	35.5	36.0	36.5	37.0	37.5	38.0	38.5	39.0	39.5	40.0	40.5	41.0
15 yrs 0 mths	31.5	32.0	32.5	33.0	33.5	34.0	34.5	35.0	35.5	36.0	36.5	37.0	37.5	38.0	38.5	39.0	39.5	40.0	40.5	41.0	41.5
15 yrs 3 mths	32.0	32.5	33.0	33.5	34.0	34.5	35.0	35.5	36.0	36.5	37.0	37.5	38.0	38.5	39.0	39.5	40.0	40.5	41.0	41.5	42.0
15 yrs 6 mths	32.0	32.5	33.0	33.5	34.0	34.5	35.0	35.5	36.0	36.5	37.0	37.5	38.0	38.5	39.0	39.5	40.0	40.5	41.0	41.5	42.0
15 yrs 9 mths	32.5	33.0	33.5	34.0	34.5	35.0	35.5	36.0	36.5	37.0	37.5	38.0	38.5	39.0	39.5	40.0	40.5	41.0	41.5	42.0	42.5
16 yrs 0 mths	33.0	33.5	34.0	34.5	35.0	35.5	36.0	36.5	37.0	37.5	38.0	38.5	39.0	39.5	40.0	40.5	41.0	41.5	42.0	42.5	43.0
17 yrs 0 mths	33.0	33.5	34.0	34.5	35.0	35.5	36.0	36.5	37.0	37.5	38.0	38.5	39.0	39.5	40.0	40.5	41.0	41.5	42.0	42.5	43.5
18 yrs 0 mths	33.0	34.0	34.5	35.0	35.5	36.0	36.5	37.0	37.5	38.0	38.5	39.0	40.0	40.5	41.0	41.5	42.0	42.5	43.5	44.0	44.5

GIRLS

GIRLS	148 cm	149 cm	150 cm	151 cm	152 cm	153 cm	154 cm	155 cm	156 cm	157 cm	158 cm	159 cm	160 cm	161 cm	162 cm	163 cm	164 cm	165 cm	166 cm	167 cm	168 cm
10 yrs 0 mths	35.0	35.5	36.0	36.5	37.0	37.5	38.0	38.5	39.0	39.5	40.0	40.5	41.0	41.5	42.0	42.5	43.0	43.5	44.0	44.5	45.0
10 yrs 3 mths	35.5	36.0	36.5	37.0	37.5	38.0	38.5	39.0	39.5	40.0	40.5	41.0	41.5	42.0	42.5	43.0	43.5	44.0	44.5	45.0	45.5
10 yrs 6 mths	36.0	36.5	37.0	37.5	38.0	38.5	39.0	39.5	40.0	40.5	41.0	41.5	42.0	42.5	43.0	43.5	44.0	44.5	45.0	45.5	46.0
10 yrs 9 mths	36.0	36.5	37.0	37.5	38.0	38.5	39.0	39.5	40.0	40.5	41.0	41.5	42.0	42.5	43.0	43.5	44.0	44.5	45.0	45.5	46.0
11 yrs 0 mths	36.5	37.0	37.5	38.0	38.5	39.0	39.5	40.0	40.5	41.0	41.5	42.0	42.5	43.0	43.5	44.0	44.5	45.0	45.5	46.0	47.0
11 yrs 3 mths	36.5	37.0	37.5	38.0	38.5	39.0	39.5	40.0	40.5	41.0	41.5	42.0	42.5	43.0	43.5	44.0	44.5	45.0	45.5	46.0	47.0
11 yrs 6 mths	36.5	37.0	37.5	38.0	38.5	39.0	39.5	40.0	40.5	41.0	41.5	42.0	42.5	43.0	43.5	44.0	44.5	45.0	45.5	46.0	47.0
11 yrs 9 mths	37.0	37.5	38.0	38.5	39.0	39.5	40.0	40.5	41.0	41.5	42.0	42.5	43.0	43.5	44.0	44.5	45.0	45.5	46.0	47.0	48.0
12 yrs 0 mths	37.0	37.5	38.0	38.5	39.0	39.5	40.0	40.5	41.0	41.5	42.0	42.5	43.0	43.5	44.0	44.5	45.0	45.5	46.0	47.0	48.0
12 yrs 3 mths	38.0	38.5	39.0	39.5	40.0	40.5	41.0	41.5	42.0	42.5	43.0	43.5	44.0	44.5	45.0	45.5	46.0	46.5	47.0	48.0	49.0
12 yrs 6 mths	38.5	39.0	39.5	40.0	40.5	41.0	41.5	42.0	42.5	43.0	43.5	44.0	44.5	45.0	45.5	46.0	46.5	47.0	47.5	48.0	49.0
12 yrs 9 mths	39.0	39.5	40.0	40.5	41.0	41.5	42.0	42.5	43.0	43.5	44.0	44.5	45.0	45.5	46.0	46.5	47.0	47.5	48.0	48.5	49.5
13 yrs 0 mths	39.0	40.0	40.0	40.5	41.0	41.5	42.0	42.5	43.0	43.5	44.5	44.5	45.0	45.5	46.0	46.5	47.0	47.5	48.0	49.0	50.0
13 yrs 3 mths	40.0	40.5	41.0	41.5	42.0	42.5	43.0	43.5	44.0	44.5	45.0	45.5	46.0	46.5	47.0	47.5	48.0	48.5	49.0	49.5	50.5
13 yrs 6 mths	40.0	40.5	41.0	41.5	42.0	42.5	43.0	43.5	44.0	44.5	45.0	45.5	46.0	46.5	47.0	47.5	48.0	48.5	49.0	50.0	51.0
13 yrs 9 mths	40.0	40.5	41.0	41.5	42.0	42.5	43.0	43.5	44.0	44.5	45.0	45.5	46.0	46.5	47.0	47.5	48.0	48.5	49.0	50.0	51.0
14 yrs 0 mths	41.5	42.0	42.5	43.0	43.5	44.0	44.5	45.0	45.5	46.0	46.5	47.0	47.5	48.0	48.5	49.0	49.5	50.0	50.5	51.0	52.0
14 yrs 3 mths	42.0	42.5	43.0	43.5	44.0	44.5	45.0	45.5	46.0	46.5	47.0	47.5	48.0	48.5	49.0	49.5	50.0	50.5	51.0	51.5	52.5
14 yrs 6 mths	42.5	43.0	43.5	44.0	44.5	45.0	45.5	46.0	46.5	47.0	47.5	48.0	48.5	49.0	49.5	50.0	50.5	51.0	51.5	52.0	53.0
14 yrs 9 mths	43.0	43.5	44.0	44.5	45.0	45.5	46.0	46.5	47.0	47.5	48.0	48.5	49.0	49.5	50.0	50.5	51.0	51.5	52.0	53.0	54.0
15 yrs 0 mths	43.0	43.5	44.0	44.5	45.0	45.5	46.0	46.5	47.0	47.5	48.0	48.5	49.0	49.5	50.0	50.5	51.0	51.5	52.0	53.0	54.0
15 yrs 3 mths	43.5	44.0	44.5	45.0	45.5	46.0	46.5	47.0	47.5	48.0	48.5	49.0	49.5	50.0	50.5	51.0	51.5	52.0	52.5	53.5	54.5
15 yrs 6 mths	44.0	44.5	45.0	45.5	46.0	46.5	47.0	47.5	48.0	48.5	49.0	49.5	50.0	50.5	51.0	51.5	52.0	52.5	53.0	54.0	55.5
15 yrs 9 mths	44.0	44.5	45.0	45.5	46.0	46.5	47.0	47.5	48.0	48.5	49.0	49.5	50.0	50.5	51.0	51.5	52.0	53.0	54.0	55.0	56.0
16 yrs 0 mths	44.5	45.0	45.5	46.0	46.5	47.0	47.5	48.0	48.5	49.0	49.5	50.0	50.5	51.0	51.5	52.0	52.5	53.5	54.5	55.5	56.5
17 yrs 0 mths	45.5	46.0	46.5	47.0	47.5	48.0	48.5	49.0	49.5	50.0	50.5	51.0	51.5	52.0	52.5	53.0	53.5	54.5	55.5	56.5	57.5
18 yrs 0 mths	45.0	46.0	46.5	47.0	47.5	48.0	48.5	49.0	49.5	50.0	50.5	51.0	51.5	52.0	53.0	54.0	55.0	56.0	57.0	57.5	58.0

Index